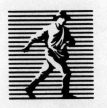

Healthy Kids for Life

Dr. Charles T. Kuntzleman

_____ SIMON AND SCHUSTER

New York ▪ London ▪ Toronto ▪ Sydney ▪ Tokyo

This book is not intended to replace the services of a physician, nor is it meant to encourage diagnosis and treatment of illness, disease, or other medical problems by the layman. Any application of the recommendations set forth in the following pages is at the reader's discretion and sole risk. If you are under a physician's care for any condition, he or she can advise you about whether the program described in this book is suitable to you.

Copyright © 1988 by Dr. Charles T. Kuntzleman

SIMON AND SCHUSTER and colophon are registered trademarks
of Simon & Schuster Inc.

Designed by Beth Tondreau Design/Jane Treuhaft
Manufactured in the United States of America

10 9 8 7 6 5 4 3 2 1

Library of Congress Cataloging-in-Publication Data
Kuntzleman, Charles T.
    Healthy kids for life/Charles T. Kuntzleman.
        p.   cm.
    Bibliography: p.
    Includes index.
    1. Physical fitness for children.   2. Children—Nutrition.
I. Title.
RJ33.K86   1988
649'.3—dc19   88-26520
                                                                      CIP

ISBN 0-671-60742-1

ACKNOWLEDGMENTS

When a book is written an author relies heavily on others. *Healthy Kids for Life* is no exception. I have many people to recognize. Larry Chilnick, of PIA Press, is acknowledged for planting the seed for this book in my mind. After my wife, Beth, and I announced our findings on children's fitness levels and heart-disease risk factors at a New York City press conference, Larry excitedly encouraged us to do a book. A book designed to help parents help make their children healthy throughout their lifetimes with wholesome family activities that are fun, meaningful, and relationship-building. Larry then connected us with Fred W. Hills, Vice President and Senior Editor at Simon and Schuster.

I extend gratitude to Fred W. Hills, and his able assistant, Jenny Cox, for patience and forcing me to include ideas that were practical and do-able for modern parents. Parents who are pulled from every angle to be "good" on the job, in the community, and at the home. Moms and dads who have genuine concern about their children but are stretched in many directions and feel overwhelmed with another responsibility.

I am grateful to Michael Boyette for his assistance in format, style, and grammar at a time when I thought this book would never get finished.

Special recognition must go to my wife, Beth, who is not only an excellent wife and mother, but a respected health and fitness professional as well. She, too, kept reminding me that this book must be based on our highly successful Feelin' Good program. A program that works, keeps fitness fun, and remembers that kids are kids— not miniature adults.

My five children, all of whom but one have left the nest, are thanked for having to endure a fitness-enthusiastic father. Deb, John, Tom, Lisa, and Becky have kept me humble, on track, and aware that fitness is only one part of a person's well-being.

Finally, my secretary, Karen Van Horn, is greatly appreciated. She has seen this manuscript at least seven times on her word processor. Karen patiently typed the manuscript, making suggestions on the book and enduring my "one more time" pleas.

To each of these terrific people: Thank you for caring and sharing.

Charles T. Kuntzleman

To Debbie Drake

The new-breed physical educator

- Dedicated to work excellence
- Committed to personal fitness
- Devoted to balanced living
- Motivated to see children achieve
- Grounded to eternal values

CONTENTS

PART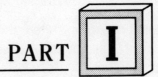

Healthy for Life

CHAPTER **1**

Healthy for Life

Are your kids in good shape? Most parents would answer yes—and chances are they'd be wrong. Consider these statistics:

- On average, today's kids get less than 15 minutes of vigorous exercise a day.
- More than 20 percent of their food calories come from sugar.
- 28 percent of them have high blood pressure.
- Almost a third have elevated levels of triglycerides.
- Nearly half of them have high levels of cholesterol—blood fats that can clog arteries and cause heart attacks.
- 68 percent eat too much salt.
- 75 percent have diets that are too rich in fat.
- 67 percent have three or more risk factors for heart disease—and virtually all have at least one risk factor.

Between 1984 and 1988 a series of studies on millions of children ages 5 to 17 have shown that 64 percent fail to meet minimum fitness criteria. Most kids reach their fitness peak—such as it is—at age 14. After that it's all downhill. The child of the eighties is less fit and more fat than the child of the sixties. Obesity is up 54 percent and superobesity as much as 98 percent. As one researcher has said, "The fattest of the fat are getting fatter faster."

Why is this happening to our kids? One factor is the schools. Surveys show that only 36 percent of America's schoolchildren have physical education every day. (This 36 percent figure may include recess.) My own research shows that in these typical physical education classes, students get only one to three minutes of sufficient exercise. Adding fuel to this dismal state of affairs is the fact that 40 percent of America's children receive physical education two or fewer times per week and only half receive instruction from qualified physical education personnel.

But there are also problems at home. The typical American diet puts us at risk for heart disease and other medical problems, and our busy, convenience-based life-style gives us too little opportunity for the kinds of activity that can keep us—and our kids—healthy and strong.

William Dietz, Jr., M.D., a pediatrician at New England Medical Center Hospitals in Boston, using data from the Health and Nutrition Examination Survey (HANES), says there is a direct relationship between a child's weight and the number of hours he or she spends watching TV. To Dietz the HANES study shows that the prevalence of obesity increases by 2 percent for each additional hour of television watched. The reasons: sitting and munching on foods high in calories, fat, and simple carbohydrates.

The program outlined in this book is based on ideas that really work. Over the past 15 years the Feelin' Good program, developed by Fitness Finders, Inc., has been used by more than 2 million kids in hundreds of communities throughout the United States and in 15 foreign countries. In developing and implementing the program, I've discovered what it takes to get kids into an exercise program and how to help them stick with it. In the pages that follow I'll share what I've learned with you to help you design a fitness program for your own family.

There are a couple of things you need to keep in mind as you use this book. First, do what works for you. Some of the suggestions in this book will click for you; others will leave you cold. Proceed accordingly. And if you get stuck, do what we experts do—improvise and use your instincts. Keep in mind that this entire process is to be fun. Don't get caught up in a drill-sergeant mentality. That will kill all interest. Stay loose. It's amazing what kids will do. Keep the pleasure part up and the "pain" part low. Participate with them and the payback to you will be as great as the benefit to your children.

Also, it's vitally important to give this program time to work. Remember, you're trying to undo years of ingrained habits. Change comes slowly at first, but I guarantee that if you can stick out the first few weeks, the program will begin to fall into place almost by itself.

The best analogy I can think of is toilet training. Unless you were one of those few parents blessed with self-training kids, I'm sure you remember how impossible those first few days (or weeks) seemed and how one day, like magic, it all came together. Well, the program you're about to embark on will be a lot easier than that and, I might add, a lost less messy.

All well and good, you may say, but your kids just aren't interested in fitness. Don't be so sure. Many parents unconsciously buy into a collection of myths about kids and fitness. Kids DO care about their bodies, fitness, exercise, and health. We think they don't because we never ask them! If your child doesn't exercise or isn't on the football team at school it doesn't mean that he doesn't care about fitness—he just hasn't been shown its brighter side. We've all had physical education teachers whose idea of punishment was 10 laps around the track; that's the kind of mentality you have to counteract with your family fitness program. Despite what those teachers led you to believe, the simple truth is that fitness can be fun. It had better be, or you'll just be wasting your time.

And finally I want to mention a benefit that goes beyond simple physical fitness—togetherness. As you go through this program you'll find yourself spending more time with your kids, talking to them, working toward common goals, and getting to know them a

---

■   ■   ■   ■   ■   ■   ■   ■   ■   ■   ■   ■

Kids and Physical Fitness

40 percent of all boys fail to pass a standard test of flexibility.

■

26 percent of the boys and 76 percent of the girls are unable to do one pull-up.

■

30 percent of the boys and 50 percent of the girls cannot run a mile in ten minutes or less.

■

28 percent are fat.

■   ■   ■   ■   ■   ■   ■   ■   ■   ■   ■   ■

---

little better. You may find out things about them that you—and they—never suspected. That's got to help you be a better parent—and it sure beats another evening in front of the television.

Behind every successful athlete there's a good coach: Vince Lombardi, Bear Bryant, Sparky Anderson. You are now going to join this august group of figures. As coach you'll be your family's fitness director, its motivator, and its strategist.

The idea of the family as a team of players will help you motivate your family to better health. This is not because you, as the coach, necessarily have any special wisdom or talent—it's simply a way to keep the program focused and moving along. You may remember those school-yard games you played as a kid and how everyone seemed to spend more time arguing than playing since nobody was in charge. That's what you want to avoid, because otherwise you'll find yourself in the middle of an empty field while your kids wander off to more promising activities.

In addition, as players family members learn to discipline themselves for the good of the team. Each encourages the others to achieve their health goals. That doesn't necessarily mean that they all have to exercise together, but it does mean that they have the responsibility to help motivate each other to walk, run, bike, or swim, and to eat right.

Remember, in your role as coach you have the biggest responsibility of all. Without your commitment, dedication, and devotion, the ideas outlined in this book simply won't work.

The first step in making your coaching plan will be a series of tests—some physical, some written—to give you an idea of your family's overall fitness. Then, using the results of this checkup, the entire family will sit down and set some goals. And then you'll embark on a two-pronged approach to fitness, through exercise and eating habits. You'll periodically evaluate your family's progress and, if necessary, set new goals.

That's actually all there is to it. As you can see, achieving fitness isn't really so formidable once you have broken it down into a series of attainable goals.

One final suggestion: After you've had a chance to explore the chapters that follow, go over your coaching plan with your family. It will help them see the overall plan, understand where they'll be going, and allay any fears that you're about to drag them into some calisthenic equivalent of Parris Island boot camp.

CHAPTER 2

The Healthy-for-Life Checkup

Before members of a team report to training camp they each get a physical from their doctor. Their coach then gives them a series of tests—for endurance, strength, and flexibility—to see if they're ready to participate in the particular sport. Our fitness checkup is similar and also has three parts: the Fitness Checkup, the Body-fat Checkup, and the Food Checkup (see pages 18 to 34).

The checkup will tell you where your family stands and where you need to begin. At the same time it will help your family start thinking in a focused way about their health and what they can do to improve it. Finally, it provides a benchmark. When you take the checkup again in a few months, you'll be able to see the progress you've made, which is a powerful motivational tool.

FITNESS CHECKUP

There are two types of physical fitness tests: performance-related and health-related. When most people (including, unfortunately, physical education teachers) talk about testing fitness, they mean performance-related fitness—areas like power, agility, balance, coordination, and reaction time. But unless your kids are headed for the major leagues, these sorts of qualities aren't all that important. You should be more concerned about the health-related aspects of fitness.

The four major health components are endurance, muscle fitness, flexibility, and body composition. Cardiovascular endurance is the ability of the body to pick up oxygen and deliver it to the muscles and other tissues. Muscle fitness is the strength and endurance of the muscles. Flexibility is the range of motion that is in the joints and limbs. Body composition refers to the ratio of fat to body weight. Endurance, muscle fitness, flexibility, and body composition can be measured respectively by the mile run, curl-ups and push-ups, the sit-and-reach test, and the skin-fold test.

These components form the basis of performance fitness. After all, an athlete lacking muscle fitness, flexibility, or cardiovascular endurance won't do well on tests measuring power, agility, or balance. And an athlete with good power but poor flexibility will be prone to injury. Similarly, athletes may show good reaction times in tests, but if they lack cardiovascular endurance, they'll tire quickly and their reaction times will slow tremendously.

But these components are important to your children's good health even if they never play sports. They improve posture, reduce the risk of premature heart disease, and result in fewer injuries, more stamina and energy, and fewer aches and pains (especially low-back pain).

Here are a few simple rules for the Fitness Checkup:

- Be sure all family members participate—including yourself.
- Encourage your kids to take all parts of the test but don't force them.
- Give them lots of praise for simply trying.
- Keep a record of the results.
- Don't compare family members.
- When you're done thank your children for their participation.

The Fitness Checkup takes about 30 minutes—more or less, depending on your family's level of fitness.

You'll need a watch with a second hand and a mat or blanket. If you're doing the checkup at home, you'll also need a cleared area at least six feet by six feet, and perhaps a space for the push-ups and curl-ups. You should also find a place to run a mile.

MEASURING ENDURANCE

I've provided four options for measuring cardiovascular fitness: the Run (see below), the Swim, the Bike Ride, or the Step Test. (See Appendix B for the swim, bike-ride, and step tests.) The run provides the best measure of cardiovascular fitness, but it also tends to be the most demanding—and if you're out of shape it can be downright grueling. So if possible let your child pick what type of test you give him. (Of course if you don't have access to a pool where you can swim laps, or if your child doesn't have a bicycle, your choices will be limited. The Step Test is good for city dwellers since it can be done in your living room. You will need a stack of newspapers to do the test.)

Test 1: The Run

First find a school track, playground, park, baseball diamond, or football field. Most tracks are a quarter mile long; four trips around make a mile. If you know that the track is 400 meters, add an extra 8 meters at the end of the last lap to make a mile. If you're not sure, give your kid the benefit of the doubt and call it a quarter mile; the 8 meters aren't all that important for our purposes anyway.

Can't find a track? Use an automobile or bicycle odometer to mark off a level one-mile route. Or use a baseball diamond; 14½ laps equal a mile. Because of the turns, times will be a little slower on a baseball diamond; also, the scenery isn't so great and it's easy to lose count of the laps. Or a football field (end zone included) may be used. Five complete circuits plus 30 yards is the equivalent of a mile.

You should run along with your child. (It's a good idea to go out beforehand and make sure you can actually run a mile. If your kids find out they can outrun you, you may get a lot of unwanted grief and teasing.)

Pace your kids, especially if they're young. Most children start this run like rabbits, only to lose steam by the end. Also, don't let them overdo it. If they can't finish the mile, simply make a note of the time and approximate distance they ran and use this as a benchmark for later runs. If you let them push themselves too far, they'll feel so lousy afterward that they'll likely be turned off to exercise for a long time to come.

As coach it's your job to make fitness a positive experience, not a punitive one. Give them lots of extra praise on this test, no matter how they do. You may want to get them running shoes, a sweatshirt, or other fitness-related gear for taking the run. Another thought is to let the kids train for two to three weeks prior to taking the test. That way they'll feel better about their performance and they won't be as sore afterward. Don't worry about the fact that you failed to get their fitness status prior to the start of the program. The point here is a positive experience, not scientific research.

TABLE 2-1 ▪ *One-Mile Walk/Run Standards for Boys*

AGE RATING	8–9	10–11	12–13	SCORE	TIME	SCORE
Excellent	<7:51	<7:50	<6:09	10		
Good	7:52–8:54	7:51–8:24	6:10–7:33	8		
Average	8:55–12:06	8:25–10:30	7:34–9:24	6		
Fair	12:07–13:52	10:31–11:10	9:25–9:59	4		
Poor	>13:53	>11:11	>10:00	2		

Note: > means "equal to or greater than." < means "equal to or less than."

TABLE 2-2 ▪ *One-Mile Walk/Run Standards for Girls*

AGE RATING	8-9	10-11	12-13	SCORE	TIME	SCORE
Excellent	<9:06	<8:56	<8.29	10		
Good	9:07-10:15	8:57-10:02	8:30-9:40	8		
Average	10:16-13:15	10:03-12:30	9:41-11:58	6		
Fair	13:16-14:53	12:31-13:14	11:59-12:48	4		
Poor	>14:54	>13:15	>12:49	2		

TABLE 2-3 ▪ *One-Half-Mile Run Standards for 6–7-Year-Olds*

RATING	Boys	Girls	SCORE	TIME	SCORE
Excellent	<4:05	<4:23	10		
Good	4:05-4:59	4:23-5:01	8		
Average	5:00-5:45	5:02-6:04	6		
Fair	5:46-6:30	6:05-6:45	4		
Poor	>6:30	>6:45	2		

MEASURING MUSCLE FITNESS

Test 2: Curl-Ups

The curl-up measures the strength and endurance of the stomach muscles. Strong abdominal muscles help prevent lower-back pain and varicose veins, flatten the tummy, and help improve posture. Tell the children:

Lie flat on your back with your knees bent and your heels 12 to 18 inches from the buttocks. Fold your arms across your chest and keep them there. Hook your toes under a desk or couch. (If you're doing this on a playground, have a partner hold down your child's feet.) First curl your head up, and then continue to curl—first your shoulders and then your back. Keep curling until your arms touch your thighs. Then uncurl until the shoulder blades touch the floor. That's one curl-up. Now do as many as you can in one minute.

TABLE 2-4 ▪ *Curl-Up Standards (number completed in one minute)*

AGE	6–7		8–9		10–11		12–13			YOUR SCORE	
RATING	M	F	M	F	M	F	M	F	SCORE	REPS.	SCORE
Excellent	36+	35+	45+	41+	48+	43+	51+	46+	5		
Good	30–35	30–34	39–44	35–40	41–47	37–42	45–50	40–45	4		
Average	19–29	19–29	28–38	24–34	31–40	28–36	34–44	29–39	3		
Fair	15–18	16–18	25–27	20–23	27–30	24–27	31–33	26–28	2		
Poor	0–14	0–15	0–24	0–19	0–26	0–23	0–30	0–25	1		

Test 3: Push-Ups (the No-Cheat, Back-Straight Military Push-Up)

Push-ups determine muscular strength and endurance of arms, shoulders, and chest. Good muscular strength and endurance of these muscles are important to help your child lift, carry, push, press, maintain good posture, and do well in sports.

For Boys Nine and Under and Girls of All Ages

- Lie on your stomach with your legs together. Place your hands so the thumbs touch the outside edge of the shoulders and the fingers point straight ahead.
- Keeping your knees on the floor (lower legs may be raised off the floor), push the upper body off the floor until the arms are completely extended. Your body should form a straight line from head to knees.

For Boys Ten Years and Older

- Lie on your stomach with your legs together. Place your hands so the thumbs touch the outside edge of the shoulders and the fingers point straight ahead.
- Keeping your toes on the floor and your legs straight, push the upper body off the floor until the arms are completely extended. Your body should form a straight line from head to toe.
- Lower your body to the starting position to complete one repetition. This exercise is to be done without resting. If you stop to rest, the test is over.
- Do as many as possible in one minute.

TABLE 2-5 ■ *Push-Up Standards (number completed)*

AGE	6–7		8–9		10–11		12–13			YOUR SCORE	
SEX	M	F	M	F	M	F	M	F	SCORE	REPS.	SCORE
RATING											
Excellent	19+	19+	20+	20+	39+	36+	41+	39+	5		
Good	14–18	14–18	16–19	16–19	31–38	31–35	35–40	32–38	4		
Average	9–13	9–13	10–15	10–15	21–30	19–30	25–34	23–31	3		
Fair	5–8	5–8	6–9	6–9	9–20	8–18	11–24	10–22	2		
Poor	0–4	0–4	0–5	0–5	0–8	0–7	0–10	0–9	1		

Why should girls do modified push-ups instead of the standard boot-camp variety? Simply because most girls lack upper-body strength. The reasons for this are partly cultural, but to a certain extent it's simply a matter of anatomy. If you ask your daughter to do regular push-ups and she can't, she may feel like a failure—and that's the last thing you want. Nonetheless, if your daughter wants to try the standard push-up, encourage her—she may surprise you. This rule also applies in reverse; if your son is over 10 and can't do a regular push-up, have him do modified push-ups. As his fitness improves he'll be able to do regular ones later on.

MEASURING FLEXIBILITY

Flexibility of the joints and elasticity of the muscles, tendons, and ligaments help prevent low back, neck, and shoulder pain, sports injuries, and soreness after exercising. It also helps improve a child's performance in all sports, and flexibility is essential for fluid, graceful movement.

Test 4: The Sit-and-Reach

The Sit-and-Reach tests the flexibility of the lower back and backs of the legs—two areas that are especially important.

You can do the Sit-and-Reach at home. If you do it at a playground, you'll need to find a wall or other flat vertical surface. Tell the test takers:

- Sit on the floor barefoot, with your legs extended. Place your heels about five inches apart, with the soles of your feet touching a wall.
- Without bending your knees, reach forward as far as possible at toe height and try to touch the wall. Bring your forehead as close to your knees as possible. Don't jerk forward; move your body only until a tug is felt.
- Hold that position and imagine the muscles relaxing.
- Stretch a little farther, until a second tug is felt. Hold for five seconds and measure how far you've reached. Try to get your palms and knuckles against the wall, fingertips touching the toes or wall, or as close to your toes as possible.

The Sit-and-Reach Test illustrates the fact that brute strength and physical fitness aren't the same. In fact, the test tends to coun-

TABLE 2-6 ■ *Sit-and-Reach Standards*

RATING	ALL AGE GROUPS	SCORE	REPS.	YOUR SCORE
Excellent	Palms flat against the wall	5		
Good	Knuckles touch the wall	4		
Average	Fingertips touch toes or wall	3		
Fair	Fingertips are 1 to 3 inches from toes	2		
Poor	Fingertips are 4 or more inches from toes	1		

terbalance the Push-Ups, since women are usually more flexible than men.

TALLYING THE RESULTS

Once your family has completed all four parts of the checkup, total the score for each participant. A score of 21 to 25 is excellent, 16 to 20 is good, 10 to 15 is average, 6 to 9 is fair, and 5 or less is poor. But keep in mind that the actual score isn't that important. Most families will probably score toward the lower end of the scale. After all, that's why you bought the book, right?

By looking at the scores in each individual category you can get an idea of the specific fitness areas that each family member should concentrate on. In Part Three I'll offer some strategies for each area. But first we have one more fitness component to measure: body-fat composition.

MEASURING BODY-FAT COMPOSITION

Measuring body fat is not simply a matter of getting on a scale. A heavy person can have very little body fat, and someone who is of average weight according to the standard height/weight charts may be carrying far too much fat. A better measure is the ratio of lean body tissue (muscles, bones, and other tissues such as the organs, nerves, and blood) to fat. Ideally, for children fat should make up only about 15 percent of total body weight.

BODY-FAT CHECKUP

This test takes about 30 minutes, and you'll need a skin-fold caliper, which you can make with tracing paper, a pencil, a thumbtack, cardboard, and an eraser. Calipers are available commercially, and range in price from $6.00 to $200. (The best for the money retails at $19.95 and can be purchased from Fitness Finders, Inc., 133 Teft Road, Spring Arbor, MI 49283.)

To make a caliper, trace the pattern on page 28 and transfer it onto the cardboard. Once the parts are cut out, a simple pivot can be made by sticking a straight pin or thumbtack through the hole marks and into the eraser.

The Skin-fold Measurement

Use the caliper to measure the back of your child's arm and his back.

Back of the Arm. Have your child stand relaxed, arms at sides. Squeeze the flesh at the back of the arm (opposite the biceps) about halfway between the elbow and shoulder. Hold the fold of flesh between the thumb and forefinger of one hand while you measure it with the caliper. (The caliper should make a slight dent in the flesh.) This can be tricky, so try a few times and figure the average.

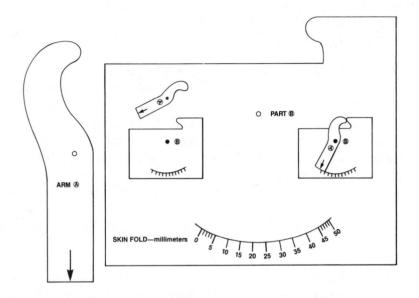

Back. Have your child stand relaxed. Measure a skin fold just below the shoulder blade. (The fold should be at a 45-degree angle to the vertical.) Again, take three measurements and figure the average.

Add the averages of the two tests, and then use Table 2-7 to find the body fat rating of your child. (Remember these are only estimates.)

TABLE 2-7 ■ *Millimeters of Fat Standards*

AGE SEX RATING	6–7 M	 F	8–9 M	 F	10–11 M	 F	12–13 M	 F	 SCORE	Mm of Fat
Excellent	9*	11*	10*	12*	10*	12*	10*	13*	5	
Good	11–12	12–14	11–13	13–15	11–12	13–16	11–12	14–16	4	
Average	13–16	15–20	14–20	16–20	13–19	17–22	13–18	17–25	3	
Fair	17–22	21–28	21–28	21–23	20–28	23–31	19–29	26–30	2	
Poor	23+	29+	29+	30+	29+	32+	30+	31+	1	

* or under

EATING HABITS

The quiz that follows will give you a good picture of your family's eating habits. Even if you think your family's diet is reasonably healthy, take the test—you may be surprised by the results.

FOOD CHECKUP
(Check Yes, Sometimes, or No)

Answer the following questions as honestly as possible. If you are not sure of an answer, quietly observe your child for a week and then answer.

1. Does your child ever eat snacks between meals?

      YES ____ SOMETIMES ____ NO ____

    If No, circle 0, check rating, and move on to   0
    Question 2.

    If Yes or Sometimes, answer the following:

    a. My child eats snacks before meals:

1. Very often (4 or more days a week)	*Circle 4*	4
2. Frequently (2 or 3 days a week)	*Circle 2*	2
3. Occasionally (1 day a week)	*Circle 1*	1

    b. My child eats snacks at bedtime:

1. Very often (6 to 7 days a week)	*Circle 3*	3
2. Frequently (4 to 5 days a week)	*Circle 2*	2
3. Occasionally (3 or less days a week)	*Circle 1*	1

Add the scores from 1, a, and b and compare to these ratings:

      Excellent   0   (Answered No to the original question)

      Good   1

Okay	2
Fair, improvement needed	3–4
Needs corrective action now	5 or more

2. Does your child eat or drink sweetened foods or beverages?

　　　YES ＿＿　SOMETIMES ＿＿　NO ＿＿

If No, circle 0, check rating, and move on to　　　　　　0
Question 3.

If Yes or Sometimes, answer the following:

a. My child drinks soda pops, "ade" type beverages, or fruit drinks:

1. Very often (5 or more times a week)	*Circle 4*	4
2. Frequently (3 or 4 times a week)	*Circle 2*	2
3. Occasionally (2 or less times a week)	*Circle 1*	1

b. My child eats candy:

1. Very often (4 or more times a week)	*Circle 4*	4
2. Frequently (2 to 3 times a week)	*Circle 2*	2
3. Occasionally (1 time a week)	*Circle 1*	1

Add the scores from 2, a, and b and compare to these ratings:

Excellent	0　(Answered No to the original question)
Good	1
Okay	2
Fair, improvement needed	3–4
Needs corrective action now	5 or more

3. Does your child eat foods that are too rich?

      YES ___ SOMETIMES ___ NO ___

If No is checked, circle 0, check rating, and move on to Question 4.

If Yes or Sometimes, answer the following:

a. My child eats ice cream and ice-cream-type treats:

1. Very often (4 or more times a week)	*Circle 4*	4
2. Frequently (2 or 3 times a week)	*Circle 2*	2
3. Occasionally (1 time a week)	*Circle 1*	1

b. My child eats pies, cakes, or cookies:

1. Very often (4 or more times a week)	*Circle 4*	4
2. Frequently (2 or 3 times a week)	*Circle 2*	2
3. Occasionally (1 time a week)	*Circle 1*	1

c. My child eats butter and/or regular margarine:

1. Very often (at each meal 4 or more days a week)	*Circle 3*	3
2. Frequently (at each meal 2 or 3 days a week)	*Circle 2*	2
3. Occasionally (at each meal one day a week)	*Circle 1*	1

Add the scores from 3, a, b, and c and compare to these ratings:

Excellent	0 (Answered No to the original question)
Good	1–2
Okay	3
Fair, improvement needed	4–5
Needs corrective action now	6 or more

4. Is your child a picky eater?

   YES ____   SOMETIMES ____   NO ____

   If No is checked, circle 0, check rating, and
   move on to Question 5.   0

   If Yes or Sometimes, answer the following:

   a. I have a difficult time getting my children
      to eat vegetables:

      1. Very often (4 or more days a week)   *Circle 3*   3

      2. Frequently (2 or 3 days a week)   *Circle 2*   2

      3. Occasionally (1 day a week)   *Circle 1*   1

   b. I have a difficult time getting my children
      to eat anything new:

      1. Very often (4 or more days a week)   *Circle 3*   3

      2. Frequently (2 to 3 days a week)   *Circle 2*   2

      3. Occasionally (1 day a week)   *Circle 1*   1

Add the scores from 4, a, and b and compare to these ratings:

Excellent	0 (Answered No to the original question)
Good	1–2
Okay	3
Fair, improvement needed	4
Needs corrective action now	5 or more

5. Is your child a fast-food/junk-food eater?

   YES ____   SOMETIMES ____   NO ____

   If you checked No, circle 0, check rating,   0
   and the quiz is completed.

If you answered Yes or Sometimes, go on to
the following:

a. My child eats at fast-food restaurants:

1. Very often (4 or more times a week)   *Circle 3*   3

2. Frequently (2 or 3 times a week)   *Circle 2*   2

3. Occasionally (1 time a week)   *Circle 1*   1

b. My child eats either crackers, pudding
pops, canned soups, gelatin-type desserts,
granola bars, packaged cereals, TV-type
dinners, potato- or cheese-type chips or
puffs, luncheon meats, etc.:

1. Very often (4 or more servings a week)   *Circle 3*   3

2. Frequently (2 to 3 servings a week)   *Circle 2*   2

3. Occasionally (1 serving a week)   *Circle 1*   1

To see how your child did in this area, add the scores from 5, a, and b
and compare to these ratings:

Excellent	0	(Answered No to the original question)
Good	1	
Okay	2	
Fair, improvement needed	3–4	
Needs corrective action now	5 or more	

This checkup is subjective. Be as honest as possible. When in doubt,
give your child the poorer score.

Look over the Food Checkup. Indicate below how your child did in the
five areas.

1. Snacking   _____

2. Sweetened foods or beverages _____

3. Rich diet   _____

4. Picky eater   _____

5. Fast-food/junk-food eater   _____

We'll come back to this later, in Chapter 10, "How to Get Your Family to Eat Right."

WHAT'S NEXT?

Okay, we've now got a handle on where your children stand in terms of fitness, fat, and food. The results of these tests provide what scientists call a baseline, an important set of numbers that lets you measure your progress. Without the baseline you have no way of knowing how far you've come or what you've accomplished.

In a few weeks you'll do the Healthy-for-Life Checkup again. Then, as now, the actual scores aren't all that important—what is important is the progress that you've made. By focusing on how far you've come rather than how far you have to go, you'll be able to give your children—and yourself—a real psychological boost.

Before you dive into the next section, take a look at your evaluation. It should give you an idea of where to start making changes. Focus on the area that needs the most improvement first, and then turn to the chapters that follow for guidelines on how to get started.

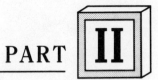

Fitness Solutions

Using the results of the tests your family completed in Chapter 2, pick the area where improvement is needed most. Then turn to the corresponding chapter in this section and get started with your family's shape-up plan.

One suggestion before you begin: Even if you're concentrating your efforts in only one area at first, look through all the chapters in this section so that you'll have an overview of where you're ultimately headed and can see how the various parts of the program fit together.

Chapter 3 offers some general guidelines about setting goals. The remaining chapters in this section each follow the same format. First there's the "theory" section, designed to give you a general overview of the subject matter. It's followed by suggestions on how to put this theory into practice—a collection of motivational tools custom-designed for kids. If your family's score in the Fitness Checkup shows that you're not quite ready to tackle a particular fitness area—or if you've decided to concentrate first on another area—a final section provides you with some simple motivational tips to help get your family started in the right direction.

CHAPTER 3

Setting Goals

Before a season begins the coach and coaching staff set goals. For example, they may say that they want to win a minimum of eight games, finish in the top ten, and/or go to a championship game. Coaches also help their athletes set individual goals, such as getting so many at-bats a season, passing 20 times a game, making 75 percent of all free throws, or running a 4:10 mile. These goals help the team and athlete set their sights on a certain level of achievement.

As you and your family set goals for your family's fitness, I recommend that you first set long-term goals (lifetime, a year, or anything in between), and then establish intermediate and short-term goals. The short-term goals should be activities that are directly under your control. For example, you may want a slimmer body (that's a general goal). Or you may be more specific and say you want to lose 25 pounds and keep the pounds off. That's a specific lifetime goal. To attain this goal you formulate a short-term goal such as "I want to lose a pound a week for the next 25 weeks." Your intermediate goal may be "At the end of three months I want to have lost twelve pounds."

The problem with these goals is that none is directly under your control. A woman's menstrual cycle, one's tendency to hold fluids, or one's muscle mass may not allow the loss of a pound a week. Or, by some quirk of your physiology, you may be able to lose only five, ten, or fifteen pounds. And if you don't lose 25 pounds, you may feel like a failure, even if you did the best your body would let you do.

To avoid the frustration establish short-term goals that are under your dominion. If you determine that you want a better-looking body, you might establish short-term goals such as: 1)Walk one to three miles a day, five days a week; 2) cut 250 calories a day from your diet; 3) learn assertiveness techniques that will allow you to express your feelings when you don't want to eat certain foods.

Your intermediate goals might be: 1) Run two to four miles a day, five days a week; 2) maintain your reduction of 250 calories a day; 3) develop assertiveness techniques; 4) learn how to cook with less fat.

In terms of specific long-term or lifetime goals, you might determine to: 1) Run from three to four miles a day and enter road races four times a year; 2) eat mostly nutritious foods, i.e., use the U.S. Dietary Guidelines; 3) continue using assertiveness techniques; 4) like your body as it is because you are doing all that is possible for it in terms of your time, ability, and goals.

THRESHOLDS

Often when people reach a goal they think the battle is over. If they slip a bit, they feel defeated and therefore soon revert to old behaviors. When setting fitness goals it's important to recognize that no one is perfect. We need flexibility for upheavals in our lives that may temporarily thwart goal-seeking.

Dr. Kelly Brownell, associate professor at the University of Pennsylvania School of Medicine and co-director of its weight-control program, illustrates this point nicely. In experiments he conducted he found it was best for dieters and exercisers to set an upper limit to what they could attain before they took action. For example, a woman had been running for six months and had worked her way up to running three to five miles a day, three days a week (her lifetime goal). She made a pact with herself that she would never miss more than three days of running in succession. If she did, she would increase the number of days the next week. In other words, she gave herself a three-day threshold, which signaled the start of corrective action.

Some examples of thresholds are:

Threshold	Corrective Action
1. No exercise for three days.	1. Ask parent to walk with me. Begin keeping a diary. Take one hour each day from watching TV to ride my bicycle.
2. Gain weight to 130 pounds.	2. Make sure I walk four times a week; food record.
3. Calorie intake level above 2,000 calories for four days a week.	3. Post weight chart on refrigerator door. Get brother to ride bicycle with me.

Thresholds such as these are important. Most people do not change their habits all at once. People fail or make small slips now and then. The thresholds permit failure without you bagging it because of indulging in a rich dessert or taking a few days off exercise.

SETTING GOALS FOR YOUR FAMILY

Now down to specific goal setting:

Step 1. Write a specific, controllable, long-term goal on a sheet of paper or a fitness card. For example:

Our Family Goal

All of us will exercise
a minimum of four times a week
(aerobically) for 30 minutes.

Save it! Review it once a week. Or post it in an obvious place.

Step 2. Now establish short-term and intermediate goals. A short-term goal might be to walk 15 minutes twice a week. An intermediate goal could be to take two 30-minute family walks a week. Also have each family member, on his own, exercise aerobically (walk, run, bike, swim, row, and/or do aerobics) for 15 minutes once a week.

Step 3. Plan ahead. You'll need to recognize obstacles and plan how to get around them. Also, determine target dates for achieving your goals and design or develop a reward for having achieved them. Record all this on a chart:

TABLE 3-1 ■ *Sample of Short-Term Goals and Problems*

SHORT-TERM GOAL	OBSTACLES	HOW TO GET AROUND THEM	DATE ACCOMPLISHED	REWARD
Family walk twice a week for 15 minutes.	Meetings, ballgames, television.	All family members agree on best time of day and which days to reserve times. Plot mileage on map.	30 days	Make up T-shirt that says, "We Did It!"

See Appendix C for short-term and long-term charts for your family. Encourage everyone to stick to the goals by doing the following.

■ *Chart progress.* Have an obvious place where family members and friends can see the progress being made. You can use a wall map or a calendar with dates designated.

■ *Commit time.* Things take on an aura of importance if they're built into your schedule. You try to be at church at a certain time and eat dinner at a certain time. Do the same with exercise. Poll the family and figure out what time is best. Everyone may need to compromise.

■ *Choose the best time.* With something like a family walk, after dinner seems best, since everyone is home. Find the time by keeping the television off for a half hour.

■ *Develop a schedule.* Don't skip all over the place with your time—morning one day, evening the next. Keep it at one particular time to build consistency and lessen the chance of forgetting.

■ *Think the part.* Have motivational posters, pictures, and/or sayings around the house. Tell everyone to think positively about exercise. No put-downs. Only positive talking and thinking.

■ *Emphasize success.* Talk about the days you've exercised, not the days you've missed. Share your success with each other and with friends.

■ *Variety.* Don't always go the same direction—take a new route. Play games as you walk. How many different smells, cars, barking dogs, or mailboxes do you see?

■ *Dress the part.* Have a walking outfit—special shoes, pants, coat, mittens—the works.

■ *Enjoy.* Don't make it punitive. Keep it fun. Don't do it because it's good for you. Do it because you like the chance to be together, to talk, to relax, to play.

■ *Don't overdo.* Exercise is pleasurable—not some masochistic event. Make haste slowly. Go at a pace and distance that is comfortable for all.

■ *Think commitment.* A commitment is a commitment, and it's intensely personal. It is your responsibility to make this decision and then put it into and keep it in practice. Once you make the decision, no excuses are permitted, except that you choose not to make a healthful change.

KEEP IT PLAYFUL

As you implement the strategies of this book and seek to get your child hooked on healthy behaviors, the key elements are your role and a playful or fun attitude.

Studies show that parents who want their kids to be in good shape should set the pace. According to Kathryn Armstrong, Coordinator of the Children in the Schools program in the Office of Disease Prevention and Health Promotion, "The kids who are the leanest and most physically fit have parents who are very active physically and watch less TV." The same can be said for their attitudes. If parents view exercise as punitive and something to prove their manhood or femininity, the kids are going to be turned off to fitness. Parents do set the tone for fitness.

It's important for parents to recognize that children want to play —just for fun. Unfortunately, 59 percent of the parents with kids in sports programs think their offspring would rather sit on the bench of a winning team than play on a losing one. Not so! say the kids. Ninety percent say playing for a losing team, rather than sitting on the bench, is best. Children like to play.

Therefore, if you have a question about what you should do, always err on the side of making fitness, good eating, and weight control fun. Keep it playful. Don't be an overzealous, pushy parent attempting to live your fitness fantasy through your children. Likewise, don't be underinvolved, uninterested, ignorant, or worried about being too enthusiastic.

CHAPTER **4**

Endurance

Endurance training—also known as cardiovascular training—is almost like a magic elixir. It helps burn off fat; it improves muscle tone; it increases the ability of the heart and arteries to supply life-giving oxygen to the body; it gives you more energy and increases your body's metabolic rate, which in turn helps you lose weight.

You can train your body to develop endurance through either aerobic or interval training. With *aerobic training* you should exercise at moderate intensity. Aerobic activities such as walking, running, biking, swimming, rope jumping, aerobic dancing, cross-country skiing, and rebounding (mini-trampolining) cause your heart to beat faster and your breathing rate to become deeper and more rapid. These exercises are considered "pay as you go." That is, they force your body to require more oxygen without producing an intolerable oxygen demand on you. Sometimes called continuous or steady-state, aerobic exercises can be done for extended periods of time—twenty minutes or longer. Aerobic exercise should not be confused with anaerobic. Anaerobic activities are intense—such as all-out sprinting. Anaerobic activities demand lots of oxygen—more than your body may be able to deliver—so you must quit the exercise in a matter of minutes or seconds.

Feelin' Good Workout

When we do a Feelin' Good gym workout with schoolchildren, we take their mental and physical characteristics into account. With popular music blaring, we start the class with walking and easy running. From there we move into rope-jumping games, aerobics, and continuous calisthenics. We avoid spending more than three to four minutes on any one of these activities. The high point of the workout is our Feelin' Good games. Here we play vigorous gymnasium video-type games that might simulate Frogger, Pac Man, Space Invaders—modifications of traditional games that maintain children's interest and enthusiasm and sport drills that are nonstop in nature. Two to three minutes are devoted to each game or activity. We conclude with a few minutes of walking and running.

Some people call Feelin' Good class "controlled chaos." I call it responding to the physical and mental characteristics of children and making sure that physical activity is fun.

Most adults like to do aerobic exercises. They enjoy logging steady-state mile after mile while running, biking, or swimming. Kids, however, struggle with aerobic exercises. Their short attention spans cause them to lose interest. Physiologically their bodies may not be able to handle one type of exercise for periods of thirty minutes or more.

Another type of endurance training is *interval training*. In intervals one vigorous exercise of about two to five minutes is followed by a comparable period of rest. This pattern of exercise-rest-exercise-rest is followed six, eight, ten, or more times. Although interval training is not as popular as aerobic training, it is just as effective (some experts say more so). Since children have shorter attention spans and may have difficulty doing an activity for a sustained period of time, they are perfect interval trainers. You may also find that it is easier to introduce children to endurance exercise by utilizing the interval training principles.

But you have to be careful. Just as a doctor prescribing medication must adjust the dosage based on such factors as the patient's age and physical condition, so you must tailor your child's exercise plan. Here's a protocol—a prescription, if you will—that you can use to determine the best kind and amount of exercise your child should be getting. It involves four factors: type of exercise, intensity of exercise, frequency of exercise, and the amount of time devoted to exercise.

THE TYPE OF EXERCISE

I polled ten fitness experts and asked them the best types of activity for improving kids' cardiovascular fitness and reducing body fat. Their favorites, in order, are as follows:

1. Cross-country skiing
2. Running
3. Swimming
4. Bicycling
5. Rowing
6. Aerobic dancing
7. Rope jumping
8. Skating
9. Walking
10. Rebounding
11. Sports (soccer, basketball, wrestling or martial arts, playing tag, sledding, racket sports)
12. Pogo stick

The first nine (cross-country skiing to walking) are excellent aerobic or steady-state exercises. The last three (rebounding, sports, and pogo stick) are best as interval exercises, although there are exceptions. For example, running can be a stop-and-go exercise (interval). That is, the child will run hard, jog, run hard, walk, etc. I've also seen kids on a pogo stick for 30 minutes with hardly a pause for station identification. In other words, they've taken an interval-type activity (pogo stick) and made it aerobic.

If the training principles outlined below are followed, any of the twelve or so activities listed above will qualify as aerobic or interval exercise. Really, the choice depends upon personal preference, as well as such considerations as your children's ages, the cost of equipment or facilities, the climate in which you live, whether the entire family can participate, and whether specialized clothing or a certain degree of skill is required.

Personally, I like running. It's simple and relatively inexpensive, and there are times when the entire family can do it together. On the other hand, many kids find running boring. (Running can be made kid-oriented by playing tag, kicking a ball on the run, creating a relay, or making up one of the hundreds of games kids have been known to create.)

Some women, I know, seem to prefer aerobic dancing. This activity can easily be steady-state or interval training, depending upon the preference of the instructor, video, or participant.

Many times kids (especially boys) will opt for sports. Sports are okay, provided that as children play, their movement is as nonstop as possible. That is, there are few time-outs, rest periods, and coaching breaks. The point is this: regardless of which of the above activities you select, the key is to keep moving (aerobic or interval) for a specified period of time at a heart rate that will elicit training of the heart and lungs.

HOW HARD? HOW MUCH? HOW OFTEN?

Once you understand the type of exercise for training, it's time to discover how hard, how much, and how often you need to exercise. Scientifically speaking, for aerobic exercise, children's heart rates must get up to 70 to 85 percent of their maximum heart rate. For interval training, they have to get up to 85 to 95 percent of their maximum heart rate with rest periods at about 60 to 70 percent of their maximum heart rates. To train their hearts children should exercise for 30 to 45 minutes four times a week. Thirty minutes is probably best. But if the kids are not pushing themselves quite as hard, it's best to extend the exercise session to 45 minutes. Exercise of this type will produce a training effect on the heart and lungs. The body is in better shape and more efficient.

To determine your child's ideal level of endurance training—aerobic or interval—begin with something called the maximum heart rate. That is the number of heartbeats per minute when your children are exercising as hard, as fast, and as long as possible. Although maximum heart rates vary from person to person, you can roughly calculate it for your child by subtracting his or her age from 220. For example, if your child is 10 years old, his maximum heart rate is approximately 210, that is, 220 − 10. (See Table 4-1, page 48.)

To figure the ideal intensity of aerobic or interval exercise, you need to know how to take your child's heart rate (see "How to Take Your Pulse," page 50). Then you can refer to Table 4-1 (see page 48) to find the range of numbers that indicates your child's ideal heart rate for exercising, either aerobic or interval.

Some people call these exercise heart rates the target exercise rate or training heart rate. No matter, it's all the same. If your child is exercising at the proper level, his heart rate during a workout will fall within the range appropriate for his or her age.

To use the Aerobic and Interval Training Chart, find your child's age in the left column. Then read the chart "mileage-map style." The first column provides your child's maximum heart rate. The second column lists the training heart-rate range if your child does steady-state or aerobic exercise. The third column indicates the training heart rate of your child, should he or she elect to do interval training. The fourth column is the "rest range" of interval training.

TABLE 4-1 ■ *Aerobic and Interval Training Chart*

AGE	I MAXIMUM HR	II AEROBIC RANGE	III INTERVAL RANGE	IV REST RANGE
6	214	150–182	182–203	128–150
7	213	149–181	181–202	128–149
8	212	148–180	180–201	127–148
9	211	148–179	179–200	127–148
10	210	147–178	178–200	126–147
11	209	146–178	178–198	125–146
12	208	146–177	177–198	125–146
13	207	145–176	176–197	124–145

If you want to check how I arrived at these figures, simply find your child's maximum heart rate in Column I. Then multiply your child's maximum heart rate by 70 percent (.70) and 85 percent (.85) for aerobic exercise. For interval training, you do a multiplication of 85 percent (.85) to 95 percent (.95). The rest range is based on 60 to 70 percent. Just remember: The aerobic exercise is steady at a heart rate of 70 to 85 percent of maximum heart rate for 20 to 45 minutes. The interval exercise is hard for two to five minutes at a heart rate of 85 to 95 percent of maximum, followed by a "rest" (easy exercise) at a heart rate of 60 to 70 percent of maximum for two to five minutes. The pattern of hard-and-easy is followed until your child gets 20 to 45 minutes of total exercise (hard and easy).

That's the theory. No self-respecting child, however, is going to let you chase after him to check his heart rate every five minutes to see if he is exercising in the proper range. Nor will the average ten-year-old stop riding his bike, jumping on his pogo stick, or playing basketball to check his pulse rate to see how he is doing. Besides, most children ten and under are unable to count their heart rates accurately.

For children, exercise and play can, and should, be synonymous. Checking heart rates distracts from the play aspect. My suggestion (commandment, actually), therefore, is to get the kids to move their bodies regularly with an eye toward having fun—not maximum heart rates and counting heartbeats.

To do the casual approach encourage your child to do one of the aerobic exercises described on page 45. Watch your child carefully. If his breathing is deeper and harder—maybe double the normal rate—he is probably okay. If you are unsure, you may want to check his heart rate on occasion. If it is in the range we just described for aerobic or interval exercise, you can conclude that his exercise level is sufficient. If you find that it is below the range, encourage your child to move more next time, to push a little harder. If it exceeds that range, you can tell him or her to back off a bit.

The substantial increase in depth and rate of breathing is a valid concept. Don't get hung up on pulse checks. Besides, you'll be amazed, as most people are, that as children run, bike, swim, etc., their heart rates usually get into the so-called training zone. Also, the more kids exercise, the more they push themselves toward the training zone.

To sum up: To be effective your child's aerobic or interval exercise sessions must be done regularly and for a sufficient length of time. Keep these guidelines in mind:

▪ To improve physical fitness your child should exercise for at least 15 minutes (preferably 20) three times a week, at evenly spaced intervals. (The exercise, of course, should be at the level that increases the depth and rate of breathing as described in the preceding section.)

■ ■ ■ ■ ■ ■ ■ ■ ■ ■ ■ ■

How to Take Your Pulse

Pulse (or heart) rate is the number of times your heart pumps blood each minute.

■

To feel your pulse, turn the palm of your hand up and place two or three fingers of your right hand on the thumb side of your left wrist. This point is called the radial pulse.

■

Sit quietly for three to five minutes, practicing taking your pulse rate. You should feel a push or thump against your fingers. Each push is one heartbeat or pulse. The number of pushes each minute is your pulse rate.

■

When you think you've got it, look at the second hand on your watch. Start at zero and count the number of heart-beats for a 6-second interval.

■

Multiply that number by 10 and you have your resting heart rate.

■   ■   ■

A normal heart rate for a child who has been sitting quietly is 72 to 110 beats per minute. For adults it is 50 to 82. (Children under 10 often have resting heart rates of 86 to 100 or higher. You'll need to check their pulse rates.)

■ ■ ■ ■ ■ ■ ■ ■ ■ ■ ■ ■

- To reduce weight or body fat he or she should work out for at least 30 minutes four times a week with a faster and deeper breathing rate.
- To reduce risk factors for heart disease, he or she should exercise for 30 to 45 minutes four times a week, following the deeper, faster breathing considerations.

These are ultimate goals. Unless your children are in top physical condition, their bodies need to adapt slowly to the overload of exercise. For unfit children, start with 10 minutes of exercise and gradually increase to the 30-minute goal.

ENDURANCE: PUTTING IT INTO PRACTICE

To get your children to undertake an aerobic or interval training program, you need to package it to increase its appeal to kids. Here are two suggested plans for an endurance shape-up program. Each of these plans has a theme, or gimmick. The idea is to have a little fun by creating some goals and rewards along the way. If you like, you can modify these plans or create your own using the same sorts of motivational strategies.

The first program outlined below is called Mileage Mania. It works best for families that don't abuse competition. If, on the other hand, your kids tend to be highly competitive, try The Equalizer—it's designed to encourage cooperation.

Mileage Mania

For this you'll need a map. On it you'll keep track of how far your family has come toward its exercise goals—literally. Every time a family member performs the exercise equivalent of walking or running a mile, he gets a one-mile credit on the map, on the way toward a particular goal.

You can play Mileage Mania in several ways. Family members can pool their mileage and chart it on a single map. This promotes a cooperative spirit, and it's also an encouragement, since mileage piles up quickly. Or, if your family prefers, each family member can chart his mileage separately—for example, by using different colors of ink. Each member can even have his own map if he wishes. If you go this route, you might need to adjust the exercise equivalents so that smaller children can keep up with their older siblings.

You can have some fun with the maps themselves too. For a family you can use a U.S. or state map; for personal mileage a state or county map is about right. Plan an interesting route, with destination points that will serve as themes for rewards.

And, of course, there's no rule that says you have to use a familiar map. You can plan a trip down the Great Wall of China or across the Andes—or even across the surface of the moon! You can take a literary trip: With younger children you might make up a scale of miles for Winnie the Pooh's Hundred Acre Woods, with a story as the reward for each milestone. For older kids use the same trick with maps taken from *The Phantom Tollbooth* or *The Hobbit*. Even better, have your kids invent their own maps, complete with their own fantasy destinations.

MILEAGE EQUIVALENTS FOR AEROBIC EXERCISE AND THE EQUALIZER

Not all children will want to run or walk. Use the following as mileage equivalents so that many activities may be placed on the map.

Activity	Mileage Equivalent
¾ mile cross-country skiing	= 1 mile
1 mile running	= 1 mile
¼ mile swimming	= 1 mile

3 miles bicycling	= 1 mile
8–12 minutes rowing	= 1 mile
8–12 minutes aerobic dancing	= 1 mile
8–12 minutes rope jumping	= 1 mile
8–12 minutes skating (ice or roller)	= 1 mile
1 mile walking	= 1 mile
8–12 minutes rebounding	= 1 mile
20 minutes sports	= 1 mile
8–12 minutes pogo stick (nonstop)	= 1 mile
20 minutes pogo stick (stop-and-go)	= 1 mile

The Equalizer

This is a simple chart to keep track of how often family members exercise. As with Mileage Mania, you should set some prearranged goals with The Equalizer. Instead of mileage, your goal would be to have each family member get a certain amount of aerobic/interval exercise (for example, 30 minutes four times a week). Every week that the family achieves this goal, they collectively earn some prearranged reward. If the family achieves the goal two weeks in a row, it earns an additional reward; for three weeks, the reward is even better, and so on.

With this system you'd assume that rewards provide the incentive. They do, but, surprisingly, so does the simple fact that you're keeping track of the amount of exercise everyone's getting. Psychological studies have shown that when you keep a chart of an activity such as exercise, it provides powerful positive reinforcement by enabling you to see how much progress you've made.

In order to minimize competition among family members, no one gets extra credit in The Equalizer. For example, if someone exercises for 60 minutes, he still gets credit only for the agreed-upon amount for exercising a certain number of times per week. This rule makes The Equalizer less intimidating, especially if one of the family members is already on a serious fitness regimen.

One of the things I like best about The Equalizer is that it encourages motivation. Little Suzy knows that if she doesn't do her part, she's not only missing out on a reward herself, but also letting down the rest of the team. In the same way she's sure to remind her big brother if he conveniently "forgets" to exercise one afternoon.

With The Equalizer, family members can agree to include sports such as basketball, dancing, fencing, field hockey, football, gymnastics (floor exercises only), ice or roller skating, ice hockey, martial arts (judo and karate), racket games (tennis, etc.), soccer, wrestling, volleyball, and even the pogo stick. But, to ensure equalization, children are to receive only half credit for participation. That means they must double the time of these sports to get full credit. That is, 40 minutes of basketball, or some similar activity, will give you 20 minutes of exercise. This allows for rest periods, coaching, and slow play.

COACHING TIP: CONTRACTS

You can adapt the idea of a contract to improve motivation in both Mileage Mania and The Equalizer, as well as in conjunction with many other coaching strategies in this book. For example, have each family member choose one fitness goal for the month, as well as a reward that he or she will earn if it's reached. Have him or her sign and date the stated goal. One or two witnesses should cosign the contract; by doing so they agree to help the contractor achieve the stated goal. (For added appeal you can buy some blank certificate paper—the kind with the fancy gold border available at an office supply store—and type or hand letter the contract on it.)

ENDURANCE TRAINING OPTIONS (FOR EXTRA MOTIVATION)

Here are some things you can do to encourage your family to exercise even if you don't adopt The Equalizer or Mileage Mania plan.

- Agree to exercise one half hour before watching TV, or just before dinner one day a week. If schedules are too complicated, set a time during the weekend.
- Have school-aged children check with the school physical education teacher regarding their participation in the President's Council on Physical Fitness and Sports Fitness Award. Kids 15 and older (including parents) can participate in the Presidential Sports Award. There are 43 qualifying sports, from archery to weight training. You select one (or more) sport and keep your own personal fitness log. For information, write:

Presidential Sports Award
PO Box 5214
FDR Post Office
New York, N.Y. 10150-5214

- **The Monster.** Once a week or month have everyone in the family get on their exercise clothing. (It's fun if everyone wears the same color T-shirt or has a similar T-shirt design.) When ready, all should run (walk when necessary) a specified distance (one to two miles is okay). An alternative is to bike six miles, walk three or swim a half mile.
- **Reward Bag or Box** (for young children). Place slips of paper with small rewards written on them in a box (a walk around the block with Mom or Dad, having a friend stay overnight, etc.). When a child does a week of exercise he or she chooses one of the activities.
- **"I Wish Book."** Each family member makes a book of rewards for himself or herself. When a goal is reached the coach chooses something from the achiever's wish book. Small children may enjoy drawing or gluing a picture on each page. This can also be done as a family activity, and special trips may be included as "wishes."
- **Birthday Walk.** Children love to do things with their parents. What better way is there to celebrate your child's birthday than to go for a walk together? You may wish to try the following:
  1. When the child turns one year old, walk one kilometer (.624 miles) together. You may have to push your child in a stroller.

If he or she can walk, you might want to walk one-fourth kilometer in the morning, one-fourth at noon, a fourth before dinner, and then another one-fourth in the evening.

2. When your child is two years old, walk two kilometers together. (Again, you may not want to do the entire two kilometers at once.)

3. When the child is three years old, walk three kilometers together.

4. Continue until your child is five, or even until he or she is 21.

To add fun to the walk, bring along a ball and kick or throw it. If you live in a cold climate, you can use shopping malls for winter walks.

- **Television Time.** If you are concerned about and want to limit the amount of television your children watch, tell them that viewing time must be earned. Establish guidelines, such as an hour of reading or studying earns a half hour of television, or an hour of active play earns a half hour of television. You may want to keep a tally sheet for each child, but be careful not to make other activities appear to be punishment. Instead, explain that you want them to enjoy some of the many other fun things to do besides watching television.

- **Something New Day.** Have family members write down an activity they would like but never have had the chance to do (i.e., hiking, bowling, and so on). Once every month or every two weeks, place the names of these activities in a hat and draw one. Plan to do this activity with the whole family.

CHAPTER 5

Muscle Fitness

Where endurance training uses activities that increase the body's ability to exercise for relatively long stretches of time, muscular fitness exercises emphasize shorter, more explosive movements. For boys, muscles are often synonymous with manliness and superhuman strength. With girls, muscles are usually not so important. In fact, many girls think that muscle fitness is unattractive—although that attitude is slowly changing.

Twenty-six percent of boys and 76 percent of girls are unable to do a single pull-up—a solid measure of muscular fitness. Unfortunately, our children's poor muscle fitness usually means they will suffer from low-back pain, an inability to meet physical emergencies adequately, and mysterious aches and pains when they become adults. Muscle fitness is essential for good health, good posture, and a good appearance.

To determine the best exercise for improving muscle fitness, I again polled the experts. Their recommendations in order of benefit: weight training (free weights and weight machines), exercise on apparatus (for example, pull-up bars), calisthenics, and partner exercises (various types of exercise that use a partner to assist). Weight-training equipment and weight machines are now available for children. If your kids are serious about training with free weights or machines, I'd consider looking into them. The new equipment is tailor-made for children's smaller, less-strong bodies.

KIDS AND WEIGHTS

I'm sure you've heard it many times: Children shouldn't lift weights because it will stunt growth. I don't know where people get the term "stunt growth." Any exercise, done improperly, can have damaging long- and short-term effects. However, we all recognize that children need to exercise their muscles.

Parents, doctors, and fitness experts encourage children to do things like pull-ups and push-ups. Then they won't let them weight train. It doesn't matter to a muscle if you exercise with your own body weight, cans of soup, or free weights.

Weight training is okay for children, but the primary concern should be safety. Before puberty children should be learning the proper technique and becoming familiar with it so they enjoy the activity.

Two or three training sessions a week is adequate. Since children have short attention spans, each session shouldn't last more than 20 minutes.

I recommend two sets of five exercises of 6 to 15 repetitions. Any five of the ten exercises listed on pages 83 to 85 may be used.

To determine the amount of weight to use at the beginning of a weight training program, take the lightest weight you have—maybe even just the bar—and put it on the floor. If your child can lift it easily, start with that weight. Tell your child to do 10 repetitions and ask how it feels. If he is grimacing by the fifth, sixth, or even tenth rep, it's too much weight. If it looks easy, add one or two pounds. Follow this pattern and the guidelines on page 59 and you will find that your kids will improve their muscle fitness very nicely.

If your child prefers calisthenics, divide his maximum effort by three and do three sets of this number. For example, if your child could do 30 push-ups in one minute, he should do three sets of 10 push-ups each during his workout (or, in training jargon, three sets of 10 reps). Again, follow the specific guidelines set forth on page 83. For other types of training, such as apparatus or partner training, I can't be as specific. Generally, I use these types of exercises as an adjunct to more specific training or for younger children.

OVERLOADING

The overload principle is the basic tenet in muscle fitness. Overloading means that when your muscles are repeatedly and regularly stimulated by a greater-than-normal weight and number of exercises, your muscles adjust and increase their capacity to perform physical work. If you want to improve your strength, your muscles must be repeatedly subjected to a training routine that stresses them more than normal. As soon as your body becomes accustomed to that exercise—that is, as soon as you no longer feel the exercise is demanding—you must increase the work (overload) so that your body is stimulated by the greater-than-normal exercise load.

COACHING TIP: DON'T PUSH IT

Children are best encouraged by watching parents exercise. They may watch for a while, jump in and exercise for five minutes, and then drop out. That's fine. The point is to encourage them, not to force them.

Be cautious with muscle fitness exercises; young children's bones, tendons, and ligaments aren't fully developed and can be damaged easily. In general, weight training is okay for kids ten and older. You can use it with younger children, provided they use light weights, get good instruction about lifting techniques, and are closely supervised, but calisthenics are usually a better choice. In any event, most kids don't get excited about weights until they're 13 or so.

One advantage of the calisthenics and partner exercises is that they are free-flowing. Many of the exercises in the next section capitalize on this fact. Whether it's utilizing ropes, tire runs, tire crawl-throughs, or moving-target throws, these exercises are particularly well suited for kids because they allow children to play spontaneously.

GETTING THE TEAM READY FOR MUSCLE FITNESS: THE HOME GYM

There are many things you can do at home to create a positive environment with respect to family fitness. The backyard is a perfect place to encourage your children to be physically fit.

Swing sets with rings and chinning bars are excellent for developing arm and shoulder muscles. The rings and the chinning bar are used for pull-up and skin-the-cat exercises. As the child develops, add gymnastic activities, like half-lever exercises, belly grinds, and birds' nests.

Ropes. From a sturdy tree limb, hang a knotted rope, three-fourths inch in diameter. Tie the first knot about four feet from the ground, spacing the rest every 12 to 18 inches apart. The knots make excellent handholds for children. When a child is first learning do not exceed three knot lengths. As he becomes more proficient, gradually increase height until he reaches 10 to 15 feet above the ground. For safety line a bed around the base of the rope with sand, pine needles, sawdust, or shavings. If the bed is long enough, it may be used for a high-jump or board-jump pit.

Tire Run. Children may run through the tires, right foot in right tire, left foot in left tire. They may try hopping from one tire to the next or hopping left and right with both feet together.

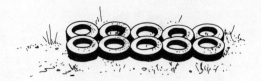

Tire Crawl-through. Partially submerge vertically 8 or 10 tires and arrange them to form a tunnel. Children may crawl through the tunnel, along the top, or whatever.

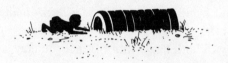

Moving-target Throw. It is best to have children throw Nerf®-type balls (football, basketball, and soccer-type ball) through the tire. Hard objects are never to be thrown because of the danger of hitting another person or object.

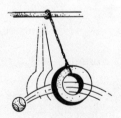

Over the Mountain. Partially submerge tires of various sizes on end, creating an incline on one side and a decline on the other, with a peak in the middle (illustration on next page).

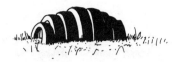

House Ladder. A ladder is an excellent device to challenge your child to be more active physically. Lean the ladder against the house, being certain that it is securely anchored. In that position, it is a substitute chinning bar. Pull-ups, knees to the chest, and half-level positions (legs raised until parallel to the ground) are a few possible ladder gymnastics.

Or place and firmly secure the ladder horizontally between two trees or some other sturdy base. Then the children can jump up and grasp a rung with both hands and advance monkey style.

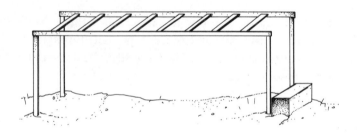

Chinning Bar. Put up chinning bars throughout the yard. They should be of varying heights for different-size children. A pipe one and three-fourths inches in diameter makes an excellent bar. For beginners, put the bar at chest height.

There are many other techniques that can be used in backyard fitness. Are you handy with tools? You can easily build equipment, such as chinning bars or a sawhorse for balancing stunts. Children also get a big kick out of jumping off objects of various heights. The pile of dirt that you just don't know what to do with, the sawhorses, a pile of railroad ties—anything of reasonable height can be used.

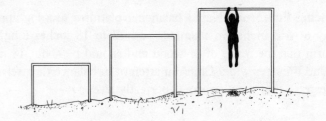

Low-level Balance Beam. Secure five 10- to 12-foot-long 2 x 4 beams (all weather treated) about six inches off the ground. Arrange a pattern with approximately one foot of space between the beams. Children can practice walking and balancing on the beams or jumping from one beam to another without fear of falling and hurting themselves.

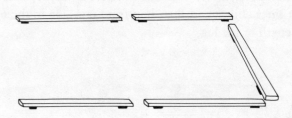

Tree-stump Steps. Secure tree stumps of various sizes in the ground, gradually increasing in height, then decreasing. Children may either hop from one stump to another or run up, then down the stumps.

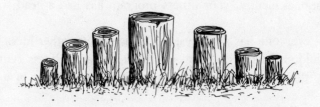

Balancing Platforms. Nail a balancing platform to a log approximately 6 to 8 inches in diameter and 12 to 18 inches long. The platform may be made of plywood and should be about 18 inches long and 6 inches wide. Children attempt to balance themselves on the beam so that the platform is perfectly level.

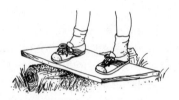

Log Hop. Arrange three logs of varying diameters parallel to each other. One activity is for children to select an appropriate-size log based on their ability and then hop from one side to the other for the full length of the log.

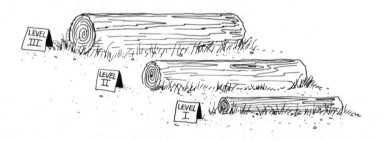

Of course if you have a swimming pool or some other elaborate recreational facility, your fitness program has had a head start already.

Not everyone has a backyard. Consider some other ideas to get the children involved. Think of the house as a fitness center. A family physical fitness room can be built or a corner of a room designated. While there is a natural tendency for mom and dad to select equipment they can use (which I discuss in Appendix D), you may want to consider equipment that makes exercise fun for children.

As you've heard throughout the book, kids see exercise as a playful, rather than a serious, pursuit. The following list includes equipment for cardiovascular and, in some cases, strengthening exercises that will show your children a good time and improve their fitness.

- Bicycles: Parents don't think of bicycles as exercise equipment, but your children's first pair of wheels will give them a good workout, and cycling never goes out of style as the younger set's most popular form of exercise. At age 10 most kids are ready for a 10-speed—the ultimate fitness toy for all ages. There are indoor bikes available for kids. Tunturi's Home Cycle is a small enough model that works well with kids and sells for $250 (see your local bicycle shop). The KidCycle, sold by Apparent, Inc., of Grass Valley, California, is for children ages 4 to 12. This glitzy bike has lights to excite kids, but the price is around $1,200.
- Mini-trampoline: What child isn't stirred by circus acrobatics. Mini-trampolines—trendy pieces of equipment—stoke the imagination and get your child hopping toward fitness (cost $59–$159). For safety, supervise your child closely. A safer version—Big Bounce—is a large inner tube with a canvas covering (cost $50).
- Pull-up bars: Hang a pull-up bar in a doorway and you will soon find your kids trying to see who can do the most. Pull-ups and flexed-arm hanging improve upper body strength and endurance. Bars run $10 to $20 and are easy to install.
- Gymboree, the pioneer of children/parent play centers, has brought their workouts into the home with a selection of wares from Gymkid (a large, multifunctional indoor play/gym set) to Gymtubes (inner tube-like inflatables for crawling through and jumping in) to Gymtracks (a balance beam with varying heights and widths). The cost for these is $10 to $150, depending upon which of the eight product lines you purchase.
- Tumbling mats, which will range anywhere from $20 to $130, depending upon the size and quality of construction.

- Pogo sticks are also a way to give kids a good workout, and if they can do it long enough, it will condition their cardiovascular system.
- Roller skates and ice skates. Skating is a type of activity that builds cardiovascular fitness and is a lot of fun.
- Jump ropes. One activity in which kids can really excel and will amaze you.

EQUIPMENT FOR YUPPY-PUPPIES

There is new equipment available that some people call "yuppy-puppy workouts." Venture Products' line of sleek kid-powered vehicles includes the Tuff Trike, an updated version of the tricycle, and the Road Rower—a vehicle that reminds me of the Irish mail (old hand-powered railroad cars)—which develops upper body strength. The Workout Wagon, a wagon in which the handle moves back and forth and gives the kids a chance to use their upper body, is also available. I find it a bit awkward, however. These items range from $150 to slightly less than $200.

Kids' weight training equipment and free weights are now available. When buying free weights for children, shop for appropriate equipment. I recommend scaled-down equipment, about 60 to 70 percent of adult size. When buying a free-weight set, choose a suitable size that grows with your children, allowing them to add plates. Hollow weights that can be filled with water, sand, or other substances are best.

American Athletic, Inc., of Jefferson, Iowa, has weight training equipment (similar to Universal equipment) made especially for prepubescent children. This equipment, called Future Force, is a 12-station total exercise system for children 8 to 15 years of age and retails for a "pricey" $7,000. Future Force equipment is recognizable by most avid body builders, offering crunch boards, high lat pull-downs, lat extensions, and the ever-present bench press.

I view the appearance of these toys as a mixed blessing. As long as they encourage play that is spontaneous and free, and not too overprogrammed by adults, they can be great. Kids should always be encouraged to exercise, but the down side is when parents start pushing kids too hard to use the equipment. If they do that, the equipment is going to collect dust, just like most parents' exercise bikes do.

To economize I suggest some of the following: Replace the weights for the exercises described on pages 86 to 89 with:

- Cans of soup—10 ounces (the original Heavy Hands®)
- Cans of fruit—1 pound
- Large cans of juice—46 ounces (almost 3 pounds)
- Books (encyclopedias)—3 to 8 pounds
- Bowling balls in a bag—8 to 16 pounds

HEALTHY-FOR-LIFE SHAPE-UP PLAN—MUSCLE FITNESS: PUTTING IT INTO PRACTICE

Motivating children under six to do specific exercises is difficult. A few get into calisthenics (maybe 5 percent) but most are not that excited. Therefore, I suggest sneaking calisthenics to kids. Some of the best tips I can give you for children of *all* ages are:

1. **Take the Test.** Once a week test the number of push-ups and curl-ups your child can do. Since progress comes quickly, this "take the test" works well for about four weeks. After that, testing once a month is better.
2. **Exercise Monopoly.** If you have Monopoly, you can adapt it to reinforce exercise concepts. Replace the names of properties with names of exercise facilities or places synonymous with fitness. Half the fun will be thinking up new names for the properties (i.e., Fred's Fantastic Fitness Facility, Boston Marathon Route). Change the "chance" cards to require participants to be active. Also, each time a person passes "Go" to

collect $200 he must do five curl-ups. The object of the game is to gain control of all the fitness facilities.

3. **Daily Exercise.** Daily Exercise is similar to The Equalizer for cardiovascular exercise. Children are given credit for doing four muscle fitness exercises four days a week. Credit is not given for more or fewer days of exercise.

4. **TV Exercise.** Commercials are a great time to do selected exercises. Most ad breaks last two minutes. Most individual ads last 30 seconds. Try to do as many repetitions of an exercise in a 30-second time span as possible. In two minutes as many as four exercises can be completed. Remember, encourage your child to vary the exercises. Switch from one body part to another. Rotate as follows: upper third, middle third, and lower third, then back to upper third, etc.

5. **Cards.** Scatter a deck of cards facedown throughout a room or play area. Have children and adults walk around the room. When you call out an exercise (curl-up, push-up, jumping jacks, etc.) each person is to go to a card, any card, and look at the face of the card. The person is to read the number on the card and do that many repetitions of the exercise. When finished the person puts the card down and proceeds to walk. A face card is equal to 10 or 15 repetitions. An ace can mean one or 20 repetitions, or no need to do the calisthenic and the chance to call out the new exercise.

6. **Musical Colors.** While music is played the children walk around colored squares of paper placed on the floor. When the music stops children move to the paper and do a specific exercise that you shout out. An alternative is to have an exercise drawn on the paper.

7. **Add an Exercise.** Get the family to stand in a circle. Have one child do an exercise of his or her choice—jumping jacks, push-ups, curl-ups, etc. The person next to him repeats the exercise twice and adds one of his own. The next person repeats each of the exercises four times and adds another, and so on around the circle. Play continues until all players have added another or until the sequence is too long to be remembered quickly.

8. **Clothespin Hunt.** Similar to an Easter egg hunt. Exercise instructions are written on index cards or pieces of paper and clothespinned in various places. Every time one is found, all family members do the exercise for 30 seconds. (Make up 20 or more cards with clothespins.)
9. **Bring Me Three.** In a park ask each child to run and find three stones (four blades of grass, two sticks, five leaves, etc.) and bring them to you. Other children do an exercise while they are running.
10. **Giant Steps and Baby Steps.** In a large area, tell children to take _____ giant steps, _____ baby steps, _____ giant steps, _____ baby steps. Go along with them around the whole play area.
11. **Copy Mommy or Daddy.** Turn on lively music (libraries have records with silly songs and music for kids). Have the child imitate Mom and/or Dad doing various exercises. Children will jump in and start exercising immediately. On occasion you may need to stop and show the children how to "get it." The typical attention span of a child is one side of an LP record.
12. **Follow the Leader, or Pied Piper.** The parent runs to a spot in the yard, park, house, or apartment and does a calisthenic exercise such as jumping jacks. Once the parent starts the exercise, the child runs to the parent and starts doing the same exercise. When the child starts the parent runs to another spot and does another exercise. The child then runs to the next spot and does the exercise the parent is doing. This pattern may be followed for 10 to 25 exercises. It may also be tied into Mileage Mania on pages 51–52. Ten to 12 minutes of Follow the Leader is the equivalent of one mile.

TRAINING PROGRAM

To read this training program answer the first question under Start (pick the appropriate age). If the answer is Yes, read to the right. If the answer is No, read downward. Follow these directions throughout.

Start   Ages 6–9

My child scored Good or   > Yes >   Congratulations! Keep up
Excellent on the Curl-Up   the good work. Encourage
Test, page 22.   your child to do the partner
        ∨   exercises: Partner Bicycle
       NO   Pumps; Partner Sit-Ups;
        ∨   Rocking Chair; Curl-Up—
                                      Push-Up; Partner V-Sit
                                      (pages 81 to 82).

My child scored Average,   > Yes >   Encourage your child to do
Fair, or Poor.   Curl-Ups three to four times
        ∨   a week. To determine how
       NO   many repetitions he or she
        ∨   should do, check the num-
                                      ber of Curl-Ups he did on
                                      the Fitness Test. Repeat
                                      that figure in one-third in-
                                      crements. For example, if he
                                      or she did 12 Curl-Ups, do
                                      four, rest a few seconds,
                                      then repeat two more times.
                                      The eventual goal for each
                                      session is 30 repetitions of
                                      Curl-Ups. To get to that
                                      goal, add a minimum of one
                                      repetition a week. Retest in
                                      six weeks.

Start   Ages 10–13

My child scored Good or   > Yes >   Congratulations: Keep up
Excellent on the Curl-Up   the good work. Encourage
Test, page 22.   your child to do the partner
        ∨   exercises: Partner Bicycle
       NO   Pumps; Partner Sit-Ups;
        ∨   Rocking Chair; Curl-Up—
                                      Push-Up; Partner V-Sit
                                      (pages 81–82). Or the fol-

lowing: Curl-Ups; Curl-Downs; Side Double-Leg Raises; Hip Lift Kicks (pages 84–85). Retest in six months.

My child scored Average.   > Yes >

V
NO
V

Encourage your child to do the following exercises three to four times a week: Curl-Ups; Curl-Downs; Side Double-Leg Raises; Hip Lift Kicks (pages 84–85). Retest in six weeks.

My child scored Fair.   > Yes >

V
NO
V

Encourage your child to do three of the following exercises three to four times a week: Curl-Ups; Curl-Downs; Side Double-Leg Raises; Hip Lift Kicks (pages 84–85). Retest in six weeks.

My child scored Poor.   > Yes >

Encourage your child to do Curl-Ups three to four times a week. To determine how many repetitions he or she should do, check the number of Curl-Ups he did on the Fitness Test. Repeat that figure in one-third increments. For example, if he or she did 12 Curl-Ups, do four, rest a few seconds, then repeat two more times. The eventual goal for each session is 30 repetitions of Curl-Ups. To get to that goal, add a minimum of one repetition a week. Retest in six weeks.

Start

Ages 6–9

My child scored Good or
Excellent on the Push-Up
Test, pp. 23–24.

\> Yes \>

Congratulations! Keep up
the good work. Encourage
your child to do a variety of
exercises, including: Partner
Wall Push-Ups; Pushing
Partners; Curl-Up—Push-
Up; Switch, Switch, Switch,
found on pages 80–83. Re-
test in six months.

V
NO
V

My child scored Average,
Fair, or Poor.

\> Yes \>

Encourage your child to do
the following exercises three
to four times a week: Partner Wall Push-Ups; Pushing
Partners; Curl-Up—Push-
Up; Switch, Switch, Switch,
found on pages 80–83. Re-
test in two months.

V
NO
V

Start

Ages 10–13

My child scored Good or
Excellent on the Push-up
Test, pages 23–24.

\> Yes \>

Congratulations! Keep up
the good work. Encourage
your child to do a variety of
exercises, including: Partner
Wall Push-Ups; Pushing
Partners; Curl-Up—Push-
Up; Switch, Switch, Switch,
found on pages 80–83. Or
do the following: Push-Ups,
High Hips; Arm Flex; Hip
Lift Kicks, on pages 83–85;
or the following: Arm Press;
Barbell Curls; Forward
Raise; French Press (pages
86–89). Retest in six
months.

V
NO
V

Start

My child scored Average.   > Yes >

       V

     NO

       V

Ages 10–13

Encourage your child to do the following exercises three to four times a week: Partner Wall Push-Ups; Pushing Partners; Curl-Up—Push-Up; Switch, Switch, Switch, found on pages 80–83. Or do the following: Push-Ups; High Hips; Arm Flex; Hip Lift Kicks, on pages 83–85; or the following: Arm Press; Barbell Curls; Forward Raise; French Press (pages 86–89). Retest in six weeks.

My child scored Fair.   > Yes >

       V

     NO

       V

Encourage your child to do the following exercises three to four times a week: Partner Wall Push-Ups; Pushing Partners; Curl-Up—Push-Up; Switch, Switch, Switch, found on pages 80–83. Or do the following: Push-Ups; High Hips; Arm Flex; Hip Lift Kicks, on pages 83–85; or the following: Arm Press; Barbell Curls; Forward Raise; French Press (pages 86–89). Retest in six weeks.

My child scored Poor.   > Yes >

Encourage your child to do Push-Ups three to four times a week. To determine how many repetitions he or she should do, check the number of Push-Ups he did on the Fitness Test. Repeat that figure in one-third increments. For example, if he is able to do 12 Push-Ups, he should do four, rest for a few seconds, then repeat two more times. The eventual goal for each session is 30 repetitions of Push-Ups. To get to that goal, add a minimum of one repetition a week. Retest in six weeks.

Family Gymnastics

These are muscle fitness activities that you can use with most children. Most can be attempted when the child is one year old. Make the activities enjoyable and they will become natural for both parent and child.

Arm Lift. Stand and face your child. Have the child extend arms up above head, with the elbows straight. Grasp the child's wrists firmly and raise the child off the floor. Keep the child rigid. Perform this exercise carefully and gradually. (Variation: Have the child grasp your thumbs, then pull the child up to shoulder level.) This exercise strengthens both the parent's and child's shoulders and upper arms.

Ball Roll. With one hand behind his or her back, the child rolls the ball in the direction you indicate: forward, backward, left, or right. The child can try this with the other hand as well. This activity improves the child's coordination and fine motor control.

Ball Under Legs. Sit facing your child, about two yards away, with your legs spread apart. Roll the ball around behind your back and under each leg, keeping the knees straight and raising the leg to pass the ball under it. Then roll the ball to your child, who repeats the exercise. This exercise improves thigh flexibility for both parent and child and also improves the child's coordination.

Bounce. Stand about two and a half yards away from your child. Bounce the ball to each other so that each can catch it without leaving his place. This develops the child's eye-hand coordination.

Bounce and Stretch. Have the child sit on the floor with legs spread. Then have the child bring the ball as high as possible over his head without lifting himself from the floor. Next the child stretches to put the ball on the floor as far in front of himself as possible. This stretches the child's lower back and shoulder muscles.

Bounce and Turn. Have the child throw the ball in the air, let it bounce once, run under it, and turn around quickly to catch the ball before it bounces again. This develops hand-eye coordination as well as body and spatial awareness.

Chase the Ball. Make a bridge with your legs. The child, from about three yards away, tries to kick the ball under the bridge. Then have the child crawl through your legs and try to catch the ball before it stops. This develops the child's foot-eye coordination as well as agility.

Crab. Have your child lie facedown on the floor. Stand behind him or her and ask the child to raise his body until his arms are straight. Then bend down and grasp your child's ankles. From here the child is to walk forward on his or her hands while you follow. This exercise strengthens the child's upper arms and shoulders.

Cradle. Have the child sit with legs crossed, holding the ankles with his hands, and then roll backward and forward on his or her back. Make sure the chin is close to the chest so that when tipped back the child's weight rests on the shoulders and not on the head. Be sure to practice on a mat or cushion. This exercise improves low-back flexibility.

Follow the Leader. Perform an activity or stunt and have the child repeat it. Then have your child perform an activity and you repeat it. This stimulates both parent and child creativity.

Foot Throw. Lying on the floor, the child is to hold a ball between his or her feet, then lift the feet quickly and release the ball so that it goes high and far. The child should aim first for distance, then for accuracy. This improves abdominal strength and aids in developing fine motor control of the muscles in the legs and feet.

Headstand. Have your child place his head on a pillow on the floor, with the rest of the body in a crouching position. Assume a kneeling position in front of the child and tell him or her to kick legs toward the ceiling for a headstand. Assist the child's movement upward, and hold the child in the position for several seconds. After a series of practices you can slowly attempt to remove your hands so that the child maintains the balance by himself. Headstands develop balance, coordination, and neck and shoulder strength.

Hop on Pop or Move on Mom. Sit on the floor with the legs spread slightly open. The child runs around your back and jumps over each leg. Now and then you should put your legs together so that the child jumps over both at once. (Variation: The child tries the same exercise with the parent's legs slightly raised.) This activity improves the child's agility as well as leg strength.

Hop Over the Stick. Move a pole or yardstick slowly back and forth, just a few inches off the floor, so your child can try to jump over it. Repeat, raising the pole a little higher. This activity strengthens the child's legs and improves coordination.

London Bridge. Have your child form a bridge by getting down on all fours and arching his or her back. Encourage your child to make the bridge very high. You are to step over the bridge several times. This activity improves the child's back flexibility and strengthens your legs.

Monkey. Stand facing your child and clasp the child's wrists. The child is to put one foot on each of your knees, then walk up your body as far as possible. To assist the child, lean backward to balance the child's weight. Then let the child walk down. This strengthens both the child's and your shoulders and upper arms.

One Bounce. The child is to throw a ball high in the air and let it bounce before he or she catches it. Eventually the child will become skilled enough so that the ball will bounce only once before being caught. This activity improves the child's eye-hand coordination and sense of timing.

Skin the Cat. Hold a pole or sturdy stick and let the child swing from it as he or she would from an exercise bar. First, the child is to try to hang only by the hands. Then he should try to hang by the hands with the knees crossed over the pole. This exercise improves arm, shoulder, and stomach strength.

Squat and Push. Face the child in a squatting position. Then, without standing up, the child tries to push you over. This activity develops balance and agility.

Step Over the Stick. The child holds a pole between both hands and steps through the triangle. He or she then steps foot by foot forward and backward without letting go of the stick. This develops shoulder flexibility.

Swan. Remove your shoes, lie flat on your back, bend your knees and draw them to your chest. Have your child place his or her abdomen on the bottom of your feet. Then hold on to the child's wrists. Slowly straighten your legs and release your hands, continuing until the legs are practically straight. The child should then extend his or her arms as in a swan dive. You should keep your hands up for protection. A more advanced skill is to do the exercise with one leg. This strengthens your stomach muscles and improves the child's balance.

Movement Exercises for Children Two and Older

Door Stand. Have the child stand on the left foot with hands on hips and right foot placed against the inside of left knee. The child should hold this position for a specified length of time and try to maintain the position with one arm in different positions—thrown across the chest, extended in front of the body, extended out to the sides at shoulder level, and so on. Then have the child switch and stand on the right foot, with the left foot placed against the inside of the right knee. Have the child repeat the exercise with eyes closed.

Stork Stand Cross. Have your child try bouncing a ball with two hands or tossing a bean bag at a target while standing in the stork stand.

Up On the Toes. Have the child stand on both feet with hands on the hips, then rise up on his toes for five or ten seconds. Repeat several times, then have the child stand on his or her toes but with eyes closed. Try this same exercise with the arms across the chest, arms out at the sides of the body, and arms extended over the head.

Balance Beam Routine. Have your child perform the following tasks on a 2 x 4 board lying flat on the floor: 1) walk the board; 2) walk sideways down the length of the board; 3) stand on toes and walk down the board; 4) try to touch his knees to the board (genuflection style) as he walks down the board; 5) walk down the board and make a 180-degree turn; 6) walk the length, complete a 180-degree turn, and then return.

Echo. Stand facing your child. Make movement (i.e., arm above head) and then have your child imitate or echo it after the first movement is completed. The movements should be fairly dynamic. After a series of movements have the child make the movements and you follow.

Energy. Stand facing your child about three to four feet away. Both your hands are to be at shoulder height, palms facing forward. Both of you are to close your eyes and turn around in place three times. Then, without opening your eyes, try to return to the original spot and position. (Variation: Use only one hand.)

Mirrored Movement. Face your child and begin moving in any way you want. Children should face you and imitate you just as if the action were being reflected in a mirror. Keep the movement slow and do not cover a great deal of floor surface.

Other Activities

Movement words are always fun. Have your child depict different types of movement. For example:

- "fast": ask child to be an arrow, a fire engine, an express train, a jet plane, a speed boat, or the wind.
- "slow": ask child to be flowers growing, a turtle, a snail, walking in snow shoes, or a big clock.
- "high": ask child to be an airplane, a kite, a stilt-walker, a clown, or a rocket ship.
- "low": ask child to be a hunter, a snake, an inch worm, a caterpillar, or a racing car.
- "strong and heavy": ask child to be a bear, a bulldozer, an elephant, a plow horse, or a train.
- "soft and light": ask child to be balloons, butterflies, feathers, elves, ghosts, or snowflakes.
- "winter": ask child to be a snowman, a snowflake, Jack Frost, the strong, cold wind, or skiing.
- "Christmas": ask child to be bells, Santa Claus, toys, excited, glad, or reverent.
- "spring": ask child to be new leaves, new flowers, warmth, prettiness, or the melting snow.

EXERCISES FOR CHILDREN SIX AND OVER

Team Up for Family Fitness

Most children love the feeling of togetherness, especially when their parents are involved. You can make fitness a family affair by buddying up with your child for partner exercises. By so doing you show your child your commitment to fitness, spend more leisure time with him or her, and encourage closeness by physical contact —especially important for men and boys in the family, who are less physically affectionate than women.

Exercising with your children is also economical because you won't need expensive equipment. Most exercises work best if partners are close in height, within five to six inches. Here are a few exercises to get you going:

Get-Up Backward. Partners stand back to back with their arms locked. Both partners gradually move the feet forward, leaning against each other until they are in a sitting position. Then, without loosening their grips, they again press against each other's backs to raise up to the starting position. This exercise works the thigh muscles.

Get-Up Forward. Partners stand facing each other, toe to toe, with hands joined. Without moving the feet or loosening their grips, partners sit down so that the thighs are parallel to the floor, then raise up again to return to the starting position. This exercise works the thigh muscles.

Tug of War. Partners stand back to back, bend over at the waist, reach between the legs and clasp one hand with the partner's hand. Each attempts to pull partner over a victory line or to the wall on his or her own side of the playing area. This exercise works the arms and shoulders.

Half-Squats. Partners stand facing each other and hold hands, then lean away from each other so that if they let go they would fall. On signal both partners bend their knees until they are parallel to the floor. Then return to a standing position. Continue until the thighs feel fatigued. This exercise works the thighs and shoulders.

Hand-Knee Lift. Partner A lies on his back with the knees bent and feet on the floor. Partner B straddles Partner A's head and places his hands on A's knees. Partner A hold's B's knees. Partner

B leans forward and A pushes B's legs up. Both participants must keep their arms stiff. This exercise works the arms and shoulders.

Partner Bicycle Pumps. Partners assume a sitting position on the floor and face one another, soles and heels of their feet touching. Partners now bicycle pump, keeping their feet in contact with one another. This exercise works the abdominal muscles.

Partner Sit-Ups. Partners assume a sitting position and face one another. The partners' legs are interlocked and they hold hands. As one partner curls upward, the other curls downward. Alternate. This exercise works the abdominal muscles.

Partner Wall Push-Ups. Ask all participants to stand with a partner approximately their own size and weight. On signal one partner begins to do wall push-ups while the other leans against his partner back-to-back. One is doing the work, the other enjoys a free ride and provides resistance. On signal they must switch positions, but in so doing they must always keep their backs together. This exercise works the upper arms and shoulders.

Pushing Partners. Partners stand facing one another with their hands on each other's shoulders. On signal each tries to push the other one backward across a designated line. This exercise works the thighs, arms, and shoulders.

Rocking Chair. Partners sit on the floor facing each other, bend the knees, and sit on each other's toes. As one partner rocks back, he or she lifts the seat of the other partner with his or her toes. Alternate. Participants must hold their partner's shoulders with stiff arms. Continue rocking back and forth. This exercise works the abdominal muscles.

Russian Kicks. Partners stand facing each other and hold hands, then lean back and adopt a crouched position with the legs bent almost 90 degrees. On signal both kick their right legs up to the right, then return them to the ground, kick their left legs up to the left and return them. Continue until the thighs feel fatigued. This exercise works the thigh muscles.

Curl-Up, Push-Up. One partner assumes a bent-knee sit-up position. The other assumes a push-up (regular or modified) position, placing hands on his partner's feet. As one partner does curl-ups, the other does push-ups. This exercise works the abdominal muscles of one partner and the upper arms and shoulders of the other. Switch roles.

Arm Pump. Stand facing one another at a distance of about three feet. Both of you are to reach forward and clasp hands, keeping your arms slightly below chest height. Alternately pump your arms back and forth while providing moderately firm resistance. This exercise conditions arm and shoulder muscles.

Leg Pump. One of you is to be on the floor with knees drawn toward your chest. The bottoms of the feet are to point toward the ceiling. Your partner is to stand facing you with feet about shoulder width apart. The standing partner should face lying partner, bend over, and place hands on partner's flexed feet. The lying partner is then to push upward with feet toward ceiling. Then return to the starting position. This exercise strengthens leg extensors.

Partner V-Sit. Sit on floor with your partner—back-to-back, upper backs pressed together and arms interlocked. From this position both of you are to raise your legs off the floor. Keep your backs straight and abdomens tight and hold legs at a 45-degree angle. Hold for specified seconds. This exercise conditions the abdominal muscles.

Switch, Switch, Switch. These exercises are designed to increase strength in a novel fashion. They are also to be performed quickly, so that pulse stays within the target heart-rate range. During these exercises one person applies resistance and the other person works against the resistance. For example:

Partner A stands with arms by his side. Partner B holds A's wrists and supplies resistance. Partner A then gradually raises his arms to shoulder height, working against B's resistance. One partner yells "Switch" every few seconds so A and B must reverse roles quickly. Other possible exercises are:

Elbow Push-Down. Partner A stands with arms extended in front, palms facing upward. He then bends his arms at his elbows. Partner B stands behind Partner A and places his hands on Partner A's elbows. Partner A gradually draws his arms backward to his waist. Partner B resists slightly.

Front Curl. Partner A stands with arms at sides, elbows bent at a 90-degree angle, palms facing upward. Partner B faces Partner A and assumes an identical position with palms facing downward and placed in hands of Partner A. Partner A curls forearms upward and Partner B resists slightly. When A's arms are brought all the way up, B pushes downward and A resists slightly.

Reverse Curl. This exercise is identical to the Front Curl, only Partner A's palms face downward.

EXERCISES FOR CHILDREN EIGHT AND OLDER

Individual Calisthenics

Here are Ten Basic Exercises. To determine the number of repetitions for each exercise, find out the maximum number of repetitions you can do in one minute and divide by three. This is the specific number of repetitions you should do three or four times.

1. Push-Ups. Lie facedown on the floor with your feet together and your hands beneath your shoulders. Keeping the body straight, extend the arms fully, then return to the starting position. This exercise helps develop the shoulders, chest, and arms.

Modified Push-Ups. Lie on your stomach with legs together. Position hands so thumbs touch the outside edges of your shoulders and fingers point straight ahead. Keeping knees on the floor and feet elevated, push upper body off the floor until arms are completely extended and you form a straight line from head to knees. Return to the starting position.

2. Curl-Ups. Lie flat on your back with the lower back touching the floor and the legs bent. Curl the head and upper part of the body upward and forward to about a 45-degree angle. At the same time contract the abdominal muscles. Return slowly to the starting position. Be certain the back is curled up so that the lower back is not aggravated. Place arms across the chest or on the thighs. This exercise is excellent for firming and strengthening the abdominal muscles.

3. One-Half Knee Bends. From a standing position, bend the knees to a 45-degree angle, with arms extended or hands on hips. Allow heels to come off the floor. Return to the starting position. This exercise strengthens the thigh muscles.

4. High Hips. Put the right hand on the floor, palm down, and keep the arm straight. Then, keeping the body rigid, extend the legs as far as they will go. The body weight rests entirely on the right foot and right hand. Now lower the hips to the floor and then raise them again as high as possible. Do these on one side and then repeat on the other side. This is a good exercise for strengthening the muscles of the arms and shoulders and for improving trunk flexibility.

5. Curl-Downs. Sit on the floor with the knees bent and the hands folded across the chest or on the ankles. Slowly lower the upper body to a 45-degree angle. Hold the position and return. This exercise strengthens the upper portion of the abdominal muscles.

6. Straddle Hops. Stand with feet together and hands on the hips. Hop off the ground so that feet are spread about three feet apart. Then return to the starting position. Continue. This exercise is a cardiovascular conditioner and strengthens the calf muscles.

7. Arm Flex. Stand with feet apart and arms extended to the sides at shoulder height. Palms should be up. Flex arms inward as though making a muscle. Touch fingertips to shoulders. This exercise strengthens the upper arms and shoulders.

8. Side Double-Leg Raises. Lie on the right side, legs extended, head supported by the right arm. Raise both legs together as high as possible, then lower to the starting position. Repeat on the opposite side. This exercise helps to firm the lateral muscles of the trunk and hips.

9. Scissors Hops. Scissors hops are similar to jumping jacks. Instead of spreading legs side to side, they move forward and back. Stand erect with hands on hips. Kick the right leg forward and the left leg backward in a scissor action. Then kick the left leg forward and the right leg backward. Keep the legs within six inches of each other. Scissors hops are a good cardiovascular exercise and strengthen the thigh and lower leg muscles. To put a little variety into the exercise, swing the arms forward and backward. When the right leg is forward, the right arm should also be forward. When the left leg is forward, the left arm should be forward.

10. Hip Lift Kicks. Sit on the floor with arms by your sides. Bend knees and place feet flat on the floor. Raise buttocks off the floor so that thighs are parallel to the floor. Kick the right leg, and then kick the left leg. Alternate kicking the right and left legs for a specified number of beats. Return to the starting position. This exercise strengthens the thighs and the shoulders.

To progressively overload your muscles with the previous ten exercises, add one repetition each week or every other week for each exercise you do.

To make this calisthenic routine more fun, turn your house into a circuit-training center with certain exercise activities performed in particular rooms of the house so that your children move from room to room. For example, let them do push-ups in the kitchen, curl-ups in the bedroom, straddle hops in the basement, and ride a stationary bicycle in the den. Give them 10 to 15 minutes to see how many times they can go through the house doing a certain number of each exercise.

EXERCISES FOR CHILDREN TEN AND OLDER

The key to a successful weight training program is allowing children to develop their interests, helping them develop some upper body strength, and making sure they do it right.

For a safe, effective program, remember the following:

- No resistance should be applied until proper form is demonstrated.
- The goal is not to see how much your child can lift. I've always believed in high reps and low weights. Children may see mom and dad lifting heavy weights and want to do the same, but children should never "max out."
- Increase weights in one- to three-pound increments after child can do 15 repetitions in good form.
- Constant supervision is absolutely necessary. Children should never be left to lift weights on their own.
- Children involved in weight training may not get stronger than other children or show immediate results. But by the time they are 15, the potential may be greater.

1. Arm Press. Develops and firms muscles of the shoulders, upper back, upper chest, and back of the upper arms. Aids in the prevention of round shoulders.

1. Stand with feet shoulder-width apart. Hold barbell in front of the chest, overhand grip, hands slightly more than shoulder-width apart.
2. Extend barbell overhead until arms are straight.
3. Return barbell to the starting position. That is one repetition.
4. Repeat.

2. **Curl-Up.** Firms the abdominal muscles.
   1. Lie flat on your back, knees bent, soles on the floor, arms folded across the chest holding a small weight (plate).
   2. Tighten your abdominal muscles and start to curl your back off the floor.
   3. Curl upward as far as possible. Return. That is one repetition.
   4. Repeat.

3. **One-Half Squat.** Develops and firms the muscles in the front of the thigh and lower leg.
   1. Stand with the feet comfortably spread.
   2. Hold the barbell in an overhand grip behind the neck, resting on the shoulders.
   3. Bend the knees to perform a half-squat (thighs no more than parallel to the floor). Return to the starting position. That is one repetition.
   4. Repeat.

4. **Barbell Curls.** Develops and firms the muscles of the upper arms and the forearms.
   1. Stand with feet apart, arms at sides. Hold the barbells against the thighs in an underhand grip.
   2. Flex forearms, raising the barbell to the shoulders.
   3. Return to the starting position. That is one repetition.
   4. Repeat.

5. **Curl-Down.** Firms the abdominal muscles.
   1. Assume a "sit-up" position, knees bent, hands placed across the chest holding a weight (plate).
   2. Slowly curl backward to a 45-degree angle.
   3. Hold this position for three seconds, or until your muscles quiver. Then return to the starting position. That is one repetition.
   4. Repeat.

6. **Lunge.** Develops and firms muscles in the front of the thigh and buttocks.

1. Stand erect, the feet together, the barbell balanced across your shoulders.
2. Take a giant step forward, bend your knees, and touch your trailing knee to the floor.
3. Push up to the starting position. That is one repetition.
4. Repeat with the opposite leg.

7. Forward Raise. Develops and firms muscles of the upper chest and shoulders.
   1. Stand with your feet waist width apart. Hold dumbbells down at the sides of your body (or resting on your thighs) in an overhand grip.
   2. Raise the dumbbells forward to shoulder height, keeping the arms straight.
   3. Lower the dumbbells to the original position. That is one repetition.
   4. Repeat.
   (Variation: Do one arm at a time.)

8. Standing Twist. Firms the muscles of the waist.
   1. Stand with your legs more than shoulder width apart, knees slightly bent.
   2. In an overhand grip, hold a weighted barbell on your shoulders, behind your head. Grip the bar near its ends, or beyond the plates, if possible.
   3. Rotate the torso slowly to one side, keeping head and knees stable. When you reach your fully twisted position, reverse. Continue alternating.
   4. Repeat. Avoid jerky movements.

9. Calf Raise. Develops and firms the muscles in the front and the back of the lower leg.
   1. Stand with the balls of the feet on a one- to two-inch block of wood or weight plate, and with the heels on the floor.
   2. Hold the barbell in an overhand grip behind the neck, resting on the shoulders.

3. Raise up on the toes as far as possible. Return to the original position. That is one repetition.
4. Repeat.

10. French Press. Develops and firms the muscles on the back of the arms and shoulders.

1. Assume a standing position with your feet shoulder width apart and your body erect. Hold a dumbbell in both hands with your arms fully extended overhead.
2. Lower the dumbbell behind your head as far as possible by bending the elbows.
3. Raise the weight back to the starting position. That is one repetition.
4. Repeat.

Remember to keep the elbows pointed straight up and close to your head throughout the movement.

Again, you're the coach. You decide which of the previous exercises are best for your family.

WEE ONE'S WORKOUT

When Dad grabs baby and lifts him over his head, he is teaching Junior the joys of fitness. Physical play, starting early in infancy, is a natural part of parent-child interaction. With the various opinions out there, parents may wonder when it is appropriate to introduce baby to a regular exercise routine.

In my opinion, it's never too early. Exercising with infants sets patterns early in life and helps your child develop physically. Before age one your baby will have a sense that exercise is a normal part of existence. If children start early and continue to exercise, by the time they are five years old it will come naturally to them.

To get your baby started on the road to fitness, follow these recommendations:

- Begin an exercise program when your baby regains his birth weight, at about one month.
- Exercise at the same time every day. You may want to make it an evening routine: exercise, bath, bottle, bed.
- Exercise in the same place every day so that baby will get used to the feeling of the floor or bed.
- Keep the temperature comfortable.
- Dress your baby in loose-fitting diapers or swimsuit, or let him exercise bare-bottom.
- Turn on music so your baby begins to associate music with exercise.

Don't force any exercise. As you move baby's arms and legs he will automatically move along. If he resists, stop.

The following exercise programs give you some basic moves appropriate to your baby's level of development. Unless otherwise indicated, perform all exercises with your baby lying face up and repeat them three to five times.

One to Two Months

Grip. Wrap your baby's hand around your forefinger, holding it in place with your thumb and third finger. Stretch out baby's arm by gently drawing the hand toward you. Do not pull the child up off the floor. Return to the starting position. Repeat five times with each arm.

Chest Cross. Using the grip that you learned in the exercise above, place your forefingers in your baby's hands. Spread baby's arms out to the side, bring them in across the chest and spread them out again. Do this exercise slowly. Repeat five times. An alternative is to move the baby's arms upward and downward.

Hamstring Stretch. Holding your baby's lower legs, gently push baby's knees up to the chest. Carefully pull the legs downward until they are fully extended. Then return to the starting position. (Often babies will instinctively kick their legs.) Repeat five times.

On the Belly. Place the baby on his or her belly and gently raise the legs. Do not cause the back to arch too much. As you raise the legs the baby will tend to rock forward.

Three to Four Months

Tug. Let the baby hold on to your fingers while you hold on to baby's hands. Pull gently on arms until upper back and shoulders arch slightly. Hold for a count of three and return to the starting position. Repeat five times.

Bicycle. Hold the baby's legs as you did for the "Hamstring Stretch." Move one leg up toward the chest while extending the other. Alternate the legs in this way, extending each leg three times. Stop and then repeat a second time. After you're done let the baby kick freely.

Nose Dive. Repeat the "On the Belly" exercise, raising the thighs higher than before. Once the thighs are all the way up, hold for a count of three seconds (1,001, 1,002, 1,003), then lower them. Do three times.

Superman. Lie on the floor with your baby resting on top of you. Baby should be lying on stomach and facing you. Hold the baby firmly by the trunk and slowly lift the baby off your chest. Talk as you do this exercise to keep the baby's attention. Repeat three to five times.

Five to Six Months

Pull-Ups. Grasp your baby as you did in the "Tug." Keeping baby's back straight, pull the baby up slowly to a sitting position. Then *slowly* and *softly* return to the floor. Repeat three to five times.

Scissors. Hold the baby's lower legs. Raise one leg perpendicular to the floor and stretch the other out parallel to the floor. DO NOT FORCE. Then alternate. Repeat three to five times.

Elbow Stand. Have baby lie on stomach. Place his or her elbows directly underneath shoulders. Grasping hips and trunk, lift baby's hindquarters up to form a 45-degree angle with the floor. Let the child rest on his or her forearms. Try to get the legs up a little higher, but make sure baby doesn't bang his nose.

Superman. See "Superman" in three- to four-month-old category.

Seven to Eight Months

Stick Rope Grip. Place a rope or a stick in front of the baby and let the child grasp it. Gently pull baby up by the rope. Return to the starting position. Repeat several times. (Be certain the child has a firm grip on the rope. Have someone behind, holding the child's back and chest, in case baby lets go.)

Toe to Ear. Bring your baby's right toe to left ear and return to the starting position. Then touch the left toe to the right ear. As you do this keep the leg straight. Repeat five times with each foot.

Wheelbarrow. Place your hands under the child's belly and pelvis, lifting the lower part of body. Baby should lift own upper weight with arms and hand. Notice that the baby will keep head upward and look forward. Hold for a slow count of three.

Superman Two. Lie flat on your back and rest your baby on your shins on his or her stomach and facing you. Start with your lower legs parallel to the floor. Pull the baby's arms out to the side, rock upward and then backward. Talk to the baby as you do the exercise.

Nine to Ten Months

Mountain Climbing. Sit on the floor. Hold the baby by his forearms and make sure that baby is also holding on to you. Let baby walk up the front of your body. This is a good exercise for baby's legs.

Crossovers. Stretch the baby's legs out straight. Cross the left leg over the right leg, touching the floor on the opposite side. Repeat with the opposite leg. Do this five times with each leg, alternating the legs.

Hand Walk. Identical to the "Wheelbarrow" except the baby walks forward on his or her own hands. Again, support baby's pelvis and trunk with your hands.

Superman Three. Lie flat. Place your feet under the baby's abdomen and raise baby up. The child should be facing you. Be certain that you hold on firmly to the child's forearms.

Eleven to Twelve Months

Rope Trick. Do this exercise over a bed and with another adult. Holding the baby's feet, let baby grip a rope. Using the rope, pull baby up slightly. Hold. After a few seconds return to starting position. It's best at this point to go to another exercise.

Handstand Stretch. Lie with your back on the floor, knees bent. With baby facing away from you and standing on your abdomen, have baby put hands on your knees. Hold baby's thighs and push them up in the air. This should be done so the baby's head is either above your knees or in between your knees. Hold for a slow count of three and then repeat three times.

More Than Just a Routine

Whether your children are doing the partner exercises, calisthenics, or weight training, you will notice that they're very enthusiastic at first, but in time they seem to become bored. It happens. Keep in mind that not all exercise programs touted for kids—whether weight training, Little League, or aerobics—address your child's psychological or even physiological needs. While some kids thrive on competition, many more do not. If you are putting undue pressure on your child, you may find that he is turned off to exercise much too soon.

Take into account the fact that children's attention spans are very short. Kids demand constant variety. They need to be entertained and have fun. Never let your children keep performing the same exercises day after day. True, kids like routine, but they also like the freeedom of change.

As your children are working out, whether on their own, with you, or with other kids, observe them. Is there enough variety? Are the children pushing? Are the children having fun? If the answer is "yes" to having fun, that will usually take care of everything. If it appears that they are just doing it to please you, you will need some serious overhauling of the program you have put together.

CHAPTER 6

Flexibility

Flexibility is what gives a dancer grace and poise. It's what gives the ballplayer that extra reach at the outfield fence. It prevents strains and other sports-related injuries. Combined with strength and endurance, flexibility provides the grace that marks the true athlete.

There are two types of exercise that promote flexibility. One is general range-of-motion exercise, which moves a limb through its full range of motion. The second is the slow, stretching exercise of yoga.

Range-of-motion exercises are probably the simplest of all exercises. To perform them, simply move each joint through its full range of motion. For example, to promote flexibility at the shoulder joint, slowly swing your arms in a 360-degree circle. Smooth rhythm is the key; there should be no jerky movements.

Once you show range-of-motion exercises to your children in an exercise session, you'll be amazed how often they'll repeat the exercises on their own. If you do these exercises once every two weeks with your kids, they will use them many more times—while watching TV, before playing games, when exercising with you, or in a pool.

RANGE-OF-MOTION EXERCISES FOR CHILDREN EIGHT AND OLDER

Alternate High-Arm Swings. Swing the arms alternately forward and back. The hands should reach at least shoulder height on the forward swing. Reach higher as progress is made. This exercise improves shoulder flexibility.

Walk—Alternate Swings. Raise both arms above the head while walking. Rotate one arm in one direction and the other in the opposite direction.

Walk—Arms Above the Head and Shoulders. Stretch the arms above the shoulders and shake them easily.

Walk—Backstroke (Backward Crawl). Alternately swing right and left arms upward, backward, and around, simulating the swimming backstroke. This exercise improves shoulder flexibility.

Walk—Cross-Body Arm Swings. Swing both arms across the body, then reverse the action by swinging both arms sideward and back as far as possible. Keep the hands chest high.

Walk—Double-Arm Pumps. Swing both arms forward and back simultaneously along the sides of the body. On the forward swings flex both arms, draw the fist in toward the shoulders, and pump twice.

Walk—Double-Arm Swings Forward and Back. Swing both arms forward and backward together while walking. As the arms swing forward they should come up alongside the ears. As they swing backward they should go slightly behind the body. This exercise improves shoulder flexibility.

Walk—Forward Crawl. When walking swing the right and left arms alternately up overhead and down in front of the body, simulating the swimming forward crawl. This exercise improves shoulder flexibility.

Walk—Giant Arm Circles Backward. Swing the arms in a complete circle, upward and across in front of the body and then backward and around. This exercise stretches and improves the flexibility of the muscles in the chest and shoulders.

Walk—High-Arm Crossovers. Reach overhead and cross the hands. Then bring the arms down alongside the body to the hips. Repeat. This exercise improves shoulder flexibility.

High-Kick Walk. Walk erect with eyes forward, chest elevated, and hands resting on hips. The toes and heels should point straight ahead. Holding the right leg stiff, kick upward, with the toe pointing toward the ceiling. Then bring the foot down alongside the body and repeat with the left leg. This exercise stretches the hamstring muscles and improves flexibility.

Straight-Leg Kick and Crossover. Perform the same motion as described for "High-Kick Walk," except this time cross the extended leg over the supporting leg and plant it on the floor. Then repeat with the other leg. This exercise improves trunk and hip flexibility and stretches the hamstring muscles.

Walk—High-Knee Action. Walk erect with eyes forward, chest elevated, and shoulders and arms in a relaxed position. Toes and heels should point straight ahead. Raise the left knee to waist height, then return it to the starting position. Then repeat with the right knee. This exercise strengthens leg muscles and improves hip flexibility.

Walk on Toes. Walk erect on the toes with good body posture. This exercise, which should always be followed by "Walk on Heels," helps to strengthen calf muscles.

Walk on Heels. Walk erect on the heels with good body posture. This exercise should always be done after walking on the toes to stretch the Achilles tendon. The exercise helps to compensate for the natural tendency for the Achilles tendon to shorten as you age and when engaged in vigorous exercise.

It's best to ease kids into stretching, e.g., during TV ads, while talking on the phone, before going out to play, and when preparing for a test.

The fluid movements of yoga are almost like ballet; they're as enjoyable to watch as they are to do. Yoga is truly an art form as well as terrific exercise for flexibility. Some people devote years to its study, but for now we'll just look at some brief samples that will promote flexibility.

Young children rarely enjoy stretching exercises unless they're in a group. You may want to explain some of the stretching exercises that follow and use them in an exercise session, working through five or ten exercises—whatever holds your children's attention. Just as with range-of-motion exercises, do these yoga-type exercises every couple of weeks or so. Then the children will tend to incorporate them whenever they exercise or see you exercising. Stretching methodology is too precise for kids under ten years of age. Some, to emulate great athletes, will do stretches, but to most kids they are a drag. Encourage your children to stretch while they watch television.

The exercises below stretch various sets of muscles, but for each the pattern is basically the same: The child should stretch until he feels a tug, hold that position briefly, and then stretch a little more. When he feels a tug again he should hold that position for ten seconds and then relax. Tell your child not to push too hard with yoga-type exercises. When he feels a tug his muscles are sending him an important signal. If he ignores it, he can injure himself.

The best time to do stretching exercises is before and after endurance exercises. Beforehand, they help warm up muscles and prevent injuries from the more taxing endurance exercises. Afterward, they help keep muscles from stiffening up. In addition, the endurance workout heats up the muscles, making them more limber for yoga-type exercises. Unfortunately the best time and when kids will stretch are worlds apart. Therefore, you will probably need to compromise with stretching while watching TV.

STRETCHES FOR CHILDREN FIVE AND OLDER

Partner Stretches

Partner Buttock Stretch. One partner lies on his back with arms by his side, knees bent. The other partner kneels and places one hand on one of the partner's knees and the other on his foot and slowly pushes the bent leg toward the shoulder. Keep the hips down. Stop when the person on the floor says to stop. Repeat for the opposite leg. This exercise stretches the gluteus muscle group.

Partner Calf Stretch. Have partners stand two or three feet apart and hold hands. Partners should then lower themselves into a squat position, using each other's hands for balance. Their seats should be close to the ground (*do not bounce*), their feet flat on the ground, and their toes pointed straight ahead. Hold and repeat. This exercise stretches the calf muscles and the Achilles tendon.

Partner Forward Tilt. One partner sits on the floor with legs crossed. The other partner stands behind and places his or her hands on the partner's shoulders. The sitting partner places his hands on the floor and walks his fingers slowly along the floor as partner assists by pushing very slightly on the shoulders and upper back. The sitting partner must look down at the floor and tell partner when to stop pushing. Change positions and repeat. This exercise stretches the lower back.

Partner Straddle Tilt. This exercise is the same as the "Partner Forward Tilt" except the partner sits with legs spread apart. This exercise stretches the lower back and inner thighs.

Partner Hamstring Stretch I. Sit on the floor with a partner. Both partners should sit facing each other with their right legs tucked in to their groins and their left legs held straight. Hold hands as one partner leans back while the other stretches forward along the right leg. Hold, then repeat for the other partner. Change positions so that the right leg is straight and repeat. This exercise stretches the muscles behind the thigh (hamstrings) as well as the low-back muscles.

Partner Hamstring Stretch II. Have partners stand and face each other. Partner A places his or her right hand on the left shoulder of B. Partner B then grasps A's right ankle and calf and gradually raises A's right leg. Partner A's leg must be held straight. Raise until A says "Stop," then hold. Repeat for the opposite leg. Switch. This exercise stretches the muscles behind the thigh (hamstrings).

Partner Lateral Stretch I. Partners stand side by side, legs one and a half times shoulder width apart. Hold the inside hands together, raise the outside hands above the head and hold. One partner leans to the left while the other partner aids the stretch by also leaning to the left and pulling. Now stretch to the opposite side. Hold. Place the opposite hand above the head and repeat. This exercise stretches the lateral muscles of the thighs.

Partner Lateral Stretch II. Partners of approximately the same height stand back to back. They should raise their arms to the sides, clasp their hands together, and place their legs one and a half times shoulder width apart. Then both partners lean to one side and hold. Repeat for the other side. This exercise stretches the lateral muscles of the thighs.

Partner Pedal Push. Partners sit facing each other, place their feet together with legs bent and hold hands. Gradually, partners raise one set of legs in unison until the legs are straight and the feet still together. Now they raise the other legs until both are straight. This exercise stretches the hamstrings.

Partner Quadricep Stretch. Partners stand side by side with inside hands on each other's shoulders to help keep their balance. Then, standing on one leg, bend the other leg and hold it by the ankle with the hand not resting on the partner's shoulder. Pull on the ankle, moving the thigh backward and stretching the quadricep muscle. Keep the thigh in close to the opposite thigh. Hold. Repeat for the other leg. This exercise stretches the muscles at the front of your thigh.

Partner Scissors. Partners stand side by side, place their inside hands on each other's near shoulder, open their legs as wide as possible, and hold in a straddle position. This exercise stretches the hamstrings.

Partner Straddle Pull. Partners sit facing each other with legs stretched as wide apart as possible and feet touching. Partners join hands and one partner leans forward as the other assists by pulling slightly and leaning back. Repeat for the other partner. This exercise stretches the inner thighs, low back, and hamstrings.

Partner Straddle Roll. This exercise is the same as "Partner Straddle Pull" except partners circle to the left slowly, then repeat to the right. This exercise stretches the hamstrings and the groin.

Roll the Ball. Give each participant a small ball or have them make a paper ball. Have them roll the ball down the right leg, then down the left leg. Open the legs wide, place the ball on the floor, roll it forward, then roll it back. Use the ball while performing a variety of stretches.

STRETCHES FOR CHILDREN EIGHT AND OLDER

Individual Stretches

Hold each stretch for five seconds. Week by week, gradually increase your holding time to 20 seconds. Instead of doing one of each, do two, holding for 20 seconds. Gradually increase your holding time. Your eventual goal: three repetitions of each stretch, holding for 15 to 30 seconds each time.

Upper Third

Elbow Special. Benefits the muscles of your chest and upper back.
1. Stand with your hands behind the head, fingers interlocked.
2. Draw your elbows back as far as possible and hold.
3. Draw the elbows forward and try to touch them together.
4. Hold and repeat.

Kneeling Shoulder Stretch. Stretches the shoulders and upper back.
1. Kneel on the floor, sit back on your heels, and look at your knees as you reach forward with your hands. Keep your seat down and continue to focus on your knees.
2. Once you have reached as far as possible, press down against the floor with your hands and you will feel your shoulders stretch.
3. Hold and repeat.

Lateral Neck Stretch. Stretches the side of the neck.
1. Lie on your back with knees bent and hands at your sides.
2. Keep the back of your head on the floor and turn your chin toward one shoulder. Make sure you keep your head on the floor.
3. Hold and repeat to the other side.

Middle Third

Knee Raises. Stretches your gluteus maximus.
1. Lie on your back with legs bent.
2. Hold the right knee with both hands and pull the knee toward your chest.
3. Hold and repeat with the left knee.

Side Stretch. Stretches the lateral muscles of your torso.
1. Stand with your feet shoulder width apart, legs straight. Place one hand on your hip and extend the other hand up over your head.
2. Bend to the side on which the hand is on the hip. Move slowly. Hold 6 to 10 seconds.
3. Repeat on the other side.

Single-Leg Tuck. Stretches the muscles at the back of your thighs (hamstrings) as well as the lower back.
1. Sit on the floor with your left leg straight and your right leg bent. Tuck your right foot into the groin.
2. Bend from the waist, reach downward, and clasp your left ankle. Pull your chest toward your left knee. Hold.
3. Repeat with the right leg.

Sitting Stretch. Benefits the muscles of the lower back and those behind the thighs (hamstrings).
1. Sit on the floor with your legs extended.
2. Bend slowly at the waist and bring your head toward the knees as close as possible. Keep your legs extended and your head down. Try to touch your toes and hold. This stretch should be done slowly.

Lower Third

Calf Stretch. Stretches the calf muscles as well as the Achilles tendon.
1. Stand with your right leg forward and your left leg back. Keep your left leg straight and bend the right leg. Keep both feet pointed straight ahead.
2. Lean forward, keeping the heel of your left foot on the ground. Hold.
3. Repeat with the right leg.

Cross-Leg Hamstring Stretch. Stretches the hamstring muscles.
1. Sit on the floor with one leg straight. Cross the other leg over the top of the straight leg. This helps stabilize the leg and prevents you from bending it during the stretch.
2. Place both hands on the straight leg and, bending slowly from the waist, walk your fingers down the leg as far as possible and hold.
3. Repeat for the other leg.

Quadricep Stretch on Side. Stretches the muscles at the front of your thighs (quadriceps).
1. Lie on your left side. Bend your right knee and hold your right ankle with your right hand.
2. Slowly pull the right leg back. Do not just pull on the foot, think of moving the entire leg. Hold.
3. Repeat for the left leg.

Sitting Groin Stretch. Stretches the muscles of your inner thighs (groin) and lower back.
1. Sit on the floor and place your heels together.
2. Grasp the inner sides of your ankles and pull your feet in toward the groin.
3. Push your knees toward the floor, using your elbows.
4. Hold, straighten legs, and repeat.

TRAINING PROGRAM ■ *Evaluating Your Children's Flexibility*

Fixing Flexibility Chart

To read this training program answer the first question under Start. If the answer is Yes, read to the right. If the answer is No, read downward. Follow these directions throughout.

Start   Ages 6–13

My child scored Good or   > Yes >   Congratulations!
Excellent on the Sit and   Keep up the good work. En-
Reach Test, pages 25–26.   courage your child to do a
            V   variety of exercises on pages
          NO   96–104. Retest in six
            V   months.

My child scored Average.   > Yes >   Have your child do four of
    V   the following stretches three
   NO   to four times a week: Part-
    V   ner Hamstring Stretch I and
II (pages 99–100), Single-
Leg Tuck, Sitting Stretch,
Knee Raises, Crossed-Leg
Hamstring Stretch, and Sit-
ting Groin Stretch (pages
102–104). Retest in 6 weeks.

My child scored Fair.   > Yes >   Have your child do three of
    V   the following exercises three
   NO   to four times a week: Part-
    V   ner Hamstring Stretch I and
II (pages 99–100), Single-
Leg Tuck, Sitting Stretch,
Knee Raises, Crossed-Leg
Hamstring Stretch, and Sit-
ting Groin Stretch (pages
102–104). Retest in six
weeks.

My child scored Poor.   > Yes >   Have your child do the Sit-
and-Reach test (pages 25–
26) three to four times a
week. Also do the Partner
Hamstring Stretch I and II
(pages 99–100). Retest in six
weeks.

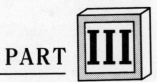

PART **III**

Training Table

CHAPTER 7

Are Our Kids "Eating to Lose"?

So far we've focused our attention almost exclusively on exercise. But that's only half the fitness equation. At least as important is the type of food your kids eat. Consider these statistics:

- 99 percent of American children eat sweet desserts at least six times a week.
- On average, they drink 24 ounces of soda pop a day.
- A third of their meals are eaten outside the home.
- Most of them have inadequate levels of fiber, vitamins, calcium, iron, or other vital nutrients in their diets.

What these and similar statistics suggest is that we're deep in the midst of a nutritional crisis in this country—a crisis that's been largely overlooked. These days consumers have more than 22,000 food products to choose from—an increase from about 6,000 in the early 1960s. Last year alone over 2,000 new products were introduced. Most of these "new and improved" products are about as healthy as the snake-oil concoctions peddled by hucksters a century ago; they're extensively processed and high in sugar, white flour, saturated fats, and salt. And they're supported by advertising campaigns costing not millions but billions of dollars.

Unfortunately, unhealthy foods happen to be profitable. Food companies know that there isn't much markup to be had on simple, fresh foods, and they know that some chocolate-coated animal-shaped breakfast cereal will win over more kids than whole wheat virtually every time. They pander to kids' still-developing tastes, loading their products with sugars and fats and using everyone from cartoon characters to comedians to sell them.

Our research shows that television advertising is second only to parental influence as a factor motivating a kid to eat or buy a certain food. Personally, I think it's immoral to make unhealthy food and then pitch it to children so shamelessly. After all, these aren't jaded consumers; selling to them is like shooting fish in a barrel—or, to use a more appropriate metaphor, like taking candy from a baby. When confronted with the best minds of Madison Avenue, kids are pretty much defenseless.

But advertising isn't the only factor contributing to our kids' bad eating habits. For a number of reasons, family eating habits have changed drastically since World War II. Most of these changes have occurred since the sixties and early seventies. Surveys show that, while there is a great interest in "healthy foods," candy and soda pop consumption are up 7.5 and 25 percent, respectively, from the years 1976 to 1981. Some experts say this trend has continued into the late 1980s. For example, one out of four three-year-olds drinks seven ounces of soft drinks every day. In addition, over 95 percent of the children fix meals and snacks, and 45 percent of all children say they would die without pizza. Going along with this trend is the fact that quality ice cream (which is exceptionally high in fat) and rich, luscious desserts such as cheesecake have increased dramatically in the past decade. For the past 20 years kids (and adults) have been fed a steady diet of sugary, fatty, salty, and cholesterol-laden foods.

Your household is not an exception. A study at the University of New Hampshire found that 25 percent of all middle-class households are child-oriented. These typical middle-class families eat to please the children, and that means sandwiches, hot dogs, and soda pop. In addition, people from smaller towns (about 30 percent of the entire population) are meat and potato eaters and are less interested in food, calories, and health. The effects of these patterns of eating show up in health tests.

THE DECLINE OF BREAKFAST

Breakfast is the most important meal of the day. After a night's sleep the body needs proteins and carbohydrates to build body tissue and provide energy. But curiously in our culture breakfast has become the most maligned meal. In many families it's nothing more than a brief snack grabbed on the way out the door to catch the bus.

If you let your kids fall into this pattern, you're asking for trouble. Consider the results of a ten-year study of school-age boys conducted at the University of Iowa. The study found that kids who skipped breakfast became careless and inattentive in the late morning. When those same boys ate a good breakfast, their schoolwork improved appreciably. In addition, some researchers believe that kids who skip breakfast are more susceptible to infection and fatigue.

Now it's true that many kids don't like breakfast. But the cause —and the cure—are simple. In most cases the problem is that breakfast comes too early in the day. If you've ever gotten up extra-early for a special meeting or trip, you know that the thought of food can be almost nauseating until you've been up and active for a while. The body simply needs time to get going in the morning, to switch over its system from the night shift to the day shift. Years ago kids often did an hour or two of chores before breakfast; these days they're often still rubbing the sleep out of their eyes when they board the school bus. If that's the case, you might consider giving your child a small nutritious snack to eat on the bus or when he or she arrives at school.

WHAT'S WRONG WITH LUNCH

The National School Lunch Act is an example of good intentions gone awry. It was established years ago when it was discovered that many kids—needy ones, especially—weren't getting enough to eat at home. Its goals were (and still are) laudable: To ensure that school-age children get at least one good meal a day and to subsidize the cost of lunch for kids from low-income families. Unfortunately, according to studies we've conducted, at least a third of all that congressionally mandated foods ends up in the trash can. The food is tasteless, unattractive, and often too greasy and salty. Our studies show that school kids are especially likely to throw out vegetables —most of which are canned—and milk, unless it's flavored with chocolate.

As troubling as it is to imagine all this food going into the Dumpster, I sometimes think it's almost as bad if the kids do eat the stuff. Most school lunches are prepared according to nutritional guidelines that were outdated 20 years ago. Sure they contain plenty of vitamins and minerals, but they're also notoriously high in fat, cholesterol, salt, sugar, and other additives. Some schools, alarmed at the food that's wasted, have taken to offering pizza and burgers prepared by fast-food restaurants. But though kids may in fact eat more of these foods than of the traditional school lunches, it's a mixed blessing—these foods usually contain excessive salt, sugar, and saturated fat.

So kids don't eat a good breakfast, they don't like lunch, and by the time they get home from school they're famished. Mom and Dad are at work, dinner isn't until seven o'clock. It's snack time.

BAD SNACKS AND GOOD SNACKS

There's nothing intrinsically wrong with a snack. Ideally, snack time could be a great time to teach children responsible eating habits. Sad to say, it doesn't usually work out that way.

Curiously, when you ask kids what their favorite snack food is, the most common response is "fruit." But if you look at what these kids actually eat for snacks, it's usually junk—candy bars, cookies, potato chips, and the like. The reason, I think, is logistics. Often fruit's not available when kids are hungry (especially if they're out of the house—when was the last time you saw a fruit vending machine?), and if it is, some preparation is often needed—peeling, cleaning, or at least rinsing. Kids can't wait; they're into immediate gratification. Add to this the ads pouring out of the television set, and you can see why healthy snacking habits break down.

Fast-food restaurants add to the snacking problem. Despite the fact that many of these restaurants now serve "healthy foods," like salads, corn on the cob, and other vegetables, the restaurant industry reports that burgers, fries, and shakes are America's top choices, day in and day out. The typical meal consumed by the fast-food feeding teenager is about 40 percent fat, 20 to 30 percent sugar, rounded off by cholesterol and sodium intakes beyond the recommended levels. Fiber intake is almost nonexistent.

Today, the increase in two-income families with less time spent in the home makes it difficult for anyone to avoid fast food. Plus, as most parents know, there is something about fast-food restaurants that is attractive—almost seductive—to kids. Children who don't eat at home wolf down a Big Mac or Chicken McNuggets. Ask a kid whether he'd rather go to McDonald's or the local Italian bistro, and Mac wins every time. Parents, as a result, frequently defer to their kids' wishes, perhaps rationalizing the situation with "At least they're eating" or "They're not wasting money on uneaten food."

It's true that it's hard to fight multimillion-dollar advertising campaigns, with their "special kid meals with prizes" and other incentives that excite children. Yet, there are things you can do to fight back. Change may not come quickly, but it is possible. A few years back, for example, a grass-roots effort by parents persuaded baby-food manufacturers to cut back on the amount of salt and sugar contained in their products. When the consumer speaks—which, unfortunately, isn't often enough—manufacturers sit up and take notice. Several years ago one major fast-food restaurant chain vowed that they would never have a salad bar in their restaurants. Technically, this is true, but they do have salads on their menus today. Consumers do have a voice. Nothing makes a company respond faster than a letter to the C.E.O.

Realistically, though, it's a lot easier to institute change at home. Unlike fitness, where your kids have to do all the work, food time is under your jurisdiction. It's never too early to begin teaching your kids to be discriminating consumers—to understand the purpose of advertising and how it works. You can also make fruit available for your kids after school and get rid of that soda bottle in the refrigerator.

And you can start to improve things at the schools. As an educator, I know firsthand that even the unreasonable demands of parents can carry great weight with principals, administrators, and school boards. So if you take the time to point out, for example, that the school lunch program is wasteful and unhealthy, you can be sure you'll be listened to. School administrators may defend the status quo at first (after all, they're only human), but if you make sure you have your facts straight and come at the topic positively—with suggestions for improvement rather than criticism alone—they'll eventually start listening to you. And remember, there is strength in numbers—even as few as two sets of concerned parents carry a lot more weight than one.

Fighting Back Against Madison Avenue

You can do more to combat bad advertising than simply teaching your kids how to recognize it. You can speak out against it. People in the ad business say that one of their greatest fears is the client who receives an irate letter. A single letter carries clout because not many people take the time to write. And advertisers and their clients are eager to know what consumers think about their efforts. So when they get a piece of evidence suggesting that their expensive efforts not only haven't worked, but have actually backfired, they take it very seriously.

CHAPTER **8**

Eating to Win

NUTRITION BASICS

No doubt you remember the Four Basic Food Groups that health teachers used to cover in grade school. You may even remember their prescription for a healthy diet. Every day, they said, you should eat four servings from the fruits and vegetables group, four from the bread and cereal group, two to three from the milk group, and two from the meat group.

Your kids are probably still hearing about the four basic food groups in school, but unfortunately the concept's become a little dated. For one thing, the foods we eat these days are anything but basic. For example, into which group does Carnation Instant Breakfast fall? How about Yoo-Hoos or Ring Dings? Tofu? More important, both nutritionists and the general public now know a lot more about what foods are good for you and bad for you. Thirty years ago you never heard about cholesterol or triglycerides, not to mention aspartame, Red Dye No. 2, monosodium glutamate, or saturated fats. So for today a better question about food is not which group it belongs in, but what's in it. Here's a brief overview of the nutrients contained in food:

Protein is the stuff of which muscles, hair, and cellular structures are made. It is essential for life. Protein's primary function is to build and repair tissue. Proteins are molecules. They are made up of amino acids linked end to end in long chains. Some experts have likened them to the cars in a long freight train. There are 20 different amino acids, as there might be 20 different freight cars. The number of each variety and the specific order in which they are linked is characteristic of each protein. The body can produce some amino acids, but not all. Essential amino acids—those which the body cannot produce—must be obtained from foods. These are called complete proteins.

The value of the protein content in food depends upon how many of the eight essential amino acids or complete proteins it contains. The best-quality protein provides the best balance of all eight amino acids. Complete proteins are found in meat, fish, poultry, eggs, and dairy products. Incomplete proteins are contained in beans, peas, nuts, breads, and cereals. They are called incomplete because they do not contain all essential amino acids. Incomplete proteins can be combined to form complete proteins. That is why vegetarians can get sufficient protein without eating animal products.

Fats are a source of energy. There are three types—saturated, unsaturated, and polyunsaturated. Saturated fats (which are a major factor in heart disease) come mostly from animals and are found in such foods as beef, pork, veal, butter, cheese, cream, milk, and shortenings. Unsaturated and polyunsaturated fats are in general much healthier, although doctors warn that too much fat of any kind may cause heart disease.

Unsaturated and polyunsaturated fats are usually derived from vegetables. They're found, for instance, in wheat germ and nuts, as well as in corn oil, safflower oil, and sunflower oil. This isn't a foolproof guide, however. Coconuts and avocados, for example, contain saturated fats. In addition, unsaturated and polyunsaturated oils may become saturated by a process of hardening called hydrogenation; that's basically how vegetable shortening and margarines are made. It's also why those ads that tout margarine made of "polyunsaturated corn oil" are misleading—even though the original oil may have been polyunsaturated, the margarine itself is

loaded with saturated fat. If the ingredients label says "hydrogenated," you know the product contains saturated fats.

When speaking of fat, cholesterol must also be considered. Many
times cholesterol is confused with saturated fat. Cholesterol is an
alcohol with fatlike properties. It is found only in animal sources of
foods, whereas saturated fats can be found in plants and animals. In
the human body about three-fourths of all cholesterol is manufactured by the liver; the rest comes from food. When the term "cholesterol" is used, it may refer to blood cholesterol, which is the
cholesterol in the bloodstream, or food cholesterol, which is the
cholesterol in our foods. The amount of cholesterol in our blood-
streams is the problematic kind.

Blood-cholesterol levels are influenced by several factors. Your
liver and intestine produce cholesterol—somewhere between 500
and 1,000 milligrams a day. This cholesterol is necessary to produce
sex hormones, transport essential fatty acids, and help form insula-
tion around the nerves. Blood-cholesterol levels are also influenced
by the kind of fat in the diet; that is, a diet high in saturated fat can
raise blood-cholesterol levels. Other factors, such as high dietary
fiber and regular aerobic exercise, can reduce cholesterol levels to a
certain degree.

The cholesterol in food also has a profound impact on blood-
cholesterol levels. The average adult male eats about 400 milligrams
of cholesterol a day. The average female eats about 265 milligrams
per day. The average child consumption is slightly less than 300
milligrams.

Fortunately, your body has a feedback mechanism that links the
amount of cholesterol it produces through the liver to the amount
of cholesterol you eat. If you eat more cholesterol, there's a tendency to produce less cholesterol by the liver. But the system works
imperfectly. If a person ate 250 to 300 milligrams of cholesterol a
day, the body would not reduce its own production. If he chose not
to eat any cholesterol at all, it would increase its production.

Studies have shown that there's a direct relationship between the
amount of cholesterol eaten and the incidence of heart disease. Researchers at the University of Minnesota and at the Harvard School

of Public Health have indicated that a diet high in cholesterol will raise blood-cholesterol levels. And while the association has not been confirmed between a high-cholesterol diet and heart disease, we do know that higher levels of blood cholesterol damage the cardiovascular system.

Historically, doctors looked at the total blood cholesterol level to determine a person's risk of heart disease. Generally, a blood cholesterol value of about 180 for adults and 140 for children was considered acceptable. Now doctors not only look at total cholesterol, they also look at the ratio of high-density lipoprotein to low-density lipoprotein. Essentially, the HDL cholesterol is the good kind, and the LDL cholesterol is the bad kind. The point is that you want to have higher levels of HDL's and lower levels of LDL's. The higher the level of HDL's, the lower your risk. It appears that if your blood cholesterol is attached to HDL rather than LDL, your blood vessels are protected rather than harmed. Exercise and perhaps some dietary programs raise HDL levels. But, again, genetics can have a profound impact on the HDL and LDL levels.

Carbohydrates, like fats, provide the body with energy. However, they're chemically less complex than fats, meaning that they tend to be consumed first and provide a source of quick fuel. (Excess calories are usually converted into fat by the body.)

There are three main types of carbohydrates: starches, sugars, and fiber. Of these, starches are the best source of energy, since starchy foods (cereals, breads, and vegetables) contain many vitamins and minerals as well as calories.

Sugar is found in many forms in a wide variety of foods. Natural sources of sugar, such as milk and fruit, are desirable for most people; concentrated sugars (cane sugar, brown sugar, syrup, and honey) tend to be high in calories and low in vitamins and minerals.

Fiber, strictly speaking, isn't a nutrient; it isn't digested by the body. Nonetheless, it offers some important benefits—by adding bulk to the diet it stimulates bowel activity and prevents constipation. It's important to eat lots of fiber if you're trying to lose weight, since it provides a feeling of fullness and increases the speed with which food travels through your digestive system (thus lowering the amount of calories that are absorbed by the body). In addition, fiber seems to have beneficial effects on the digestive tract itself. It has been shown to be useful in the treatment of diverticulosis, and diets that are low in fiber have been associated with colon cancer, diabetes, and heart disease.

The typical American diet is relatively low in fiber. While nutritionists recommend 25 grams a day of fiber, most Americans consume less than 10 grams. Our own studies have shown that young boys and girls rarely get more than four grams of fiber a day.

Minerals—substances such as iron, calcium, zinc, and magnesium—help regulate various body functions. They're also important to the development of bones and body tissues. Again, our studies have shown that most kids don't get enough of these important substances—especially iron and calcium. Iron deficiencies lead to anemia, with such symptoms as fatigue and, in teenagers and older females, menstrual irregularities. Calcium deficiencies can hinder growth and cause osteoporosis later in life.

Vitamins, like minerals, help control the body's functions; they also play an important role in energy production, normal growth, resistance to infection, and general health. There are two types of vitamins: fat-soluble (vitamins A, D, E, and K) and water-soluble vitamins (the B vitamins and vitamin C). Water-soluble vitamins must be replenished continually—the body can't store them. Fat-soluble vitamins, by contrast, are stored in body fat, but you have to be careful—since their primary source is fatty foods, supplements may be needed if fat consumption is cut drastically.

About 30 percent of America's children have deficiencies of vitamins A and C. The solution is simple: An extra carrot and a glass of orange juice provide ample quantities.

Water. You might be surprised to see water on this list, but it constitutes about 70 percent of a person's body weight, and in many ways it is the most important nutritional ingredient of all. You may be able to survive without carbohydrates, fats, proteins, vitamins, and minerals for months—in some instances for years—but without water you will only make it for about three days. Fortunately, the body's thirst mechanism does a good job of ensuring that we get adequate fluids. The trick with kids, however, is to convince them that when they're thirsty, their bodies are asking for water, not some carbonated concoction laced with sugar and caffeine.

THE EIGHT BASIC FOOD GROUPS

Armed with this more thorough knowledge of foods, we can replace the old idea of the Four Basic Foods with a new and much more useful grouping of Eight Basic Food Groups. This system classifies food according to nutritional content rather than the source of the food.

Within the Eight Basic Food Groups are two categories:

Category One: Basic Foods

    Group 1: Vegetables
    Group 2: Fruits
    Group 3: Dairy Products
    Group 4: Protein Foods
    Group 5: Bread, Cereals, and Grains
    Group 6: Vegetable Oils and Fats

Category Two: Nonbasic Foods

    Group 7: Combination/Fabricated Foods
    Group 8: Sweets, Alcohol, and Other Beverages

Vegetables. Important for normal growth, good vision, energy, and resistance to infection, vegetables are rich in vitamins, minerals, and carbohydrates. There are two basic types: starchy vegetables (primarily yellow and white vegetables) and nonstarchy vegetables, which are usually green and leafy.

The nutritional content of vegetables is very fragile and can be destroyed by improper storage and cooking. Here are some tips for selecting and cooking them in ways that preserve not only their nutrients but also their flavor:

- Select fresh vegetables (that is, right out of the garden or from the farmer) first, frozen second, fresh from the grocer's stand third, low-salt canned fourth, and normal canned fifth. If you canned your own garden-fresh vegetables, they should be selected fourth unless you salted the vegetables heavily. Then place your canned vegetables fifth.
- Cook vegetables in small quantities of water and for a short period of time. Steaming is the best method to preserve vitamins and minerals. Keep cooking vessels tightly covered and leave "skins" on vegetables whenever possible. This technique of not using much water restricts chemical reactions that may destroy some vitamins and minerals. If you do cook with large amounts of water, boil in an uncovered pot and be careful not to overcook. When vegetables are cooked a long time, don't throw the water away, save and use it as a base for soup or stew.
- Do not add soda in cooking vegetables or cook in copper containers. Alkali and copper hasten vitamin destruction.
- Do not allow "quick frozen" foods to thaw out before cooking. Place frozen vegetables directly into boiling water.
- Microwave frozen vegetables in their own bag or box following manufacturer's instructions.
- Remember, frying greatly increases fat content and calories of vegetables.
- Stir-fry or steam green vegetables.
- Allow water to boil vigorously for one minute before dumping in vegetables. (Quick boiling reduces the loss of vitamins and minerals. A recent article in *American Health* indicated that if you put cabbage in a pot of cold water and bring it to a boil, the cabbage could lose 25 percent of the vitamin C in 15 minutes. If you boil the water first, and then place the cabbage in the water, only 2 percent of the vitamin C is lost.)

If you select frozen vegetables, here are some national brands that are low in salt.

- Birds Eye Broccoli Spears
- Birds Eye Cooked Winter Squash
- Birds Eye Cut Green Beans
- Birds Eye Little Ears of Corn
- Birds Eye Sweet Corn
- Seabrook Farms Baby Brussel Sprouts

If you select canned vegetables, here are some national brands that are low in salt.

- Aunt Millie's Meatless Traditional Spaghetti Sauce—sodium, 300 mg.
- Campbell's V-8 Juice—no salt added
- Contadina Tomato Paste
- Libby's Natural Pack Mixed Vegetables
- Orville Redenbacher's Gourmet Popcorn
- Baby Food
  Beech-Nut Stage One
  Mohawk Valley Green Beans
  Gerber Strained Mixed Vegetables
  Gerber Strained Vegetables with Chicken
  Heinz Vegetables, Egg Noodles, and Chicken

Of course regional brands of frozen and canned vegetables may be equally low in salt—just be sure to check labels for comparison.

Fruits. Like vegetables, fruits are important for growth, energy, vision, healthy tissue, and resistance to infection. They're especially important as sources of vitamin A and vitamin C. And, again like veggies, the nutrients they contain are easily damaged—vitamin C in particular is easily destroyed by exposure to air and heat. To help preserve their nutritional value, try the following:

- As with vegetables, select fresh fruits (out of the garden or from the farmer) as your first choice, frozen second, fresh from the grocer's stand third, low-sugar canned fourth, and normal canned fifth. If you canned your own garden (or farmer's) fruit, they may be selected as your fourth preference, unless you laced the fruit heavily with sugar (then your canned fruit should rank as your fifth choice).

■ If you select frozen fruit, remember that Birds Eye products tend to retain significantly more natural vitamins and minerals than other brands.

■ The most popular manufacturers of canned fruits, Del Monte, Dole, and Libby, offer fruits packed in their own unsweetened juice. Select these canned products rather than those fruits packed in heavy syrup.

A few of my favorite canned fruits (they are lower in sugar and corn syrup) are Del Monte Pineapple Chunks in Pineapple Juice, Del Monte Sliced Pineapple in Pineapple Juice, Dole Pineapple Juice, Dole Sliced Pineapple in Pineapple Juice, Lucky Leaf Apple Juice, Libby's Lite Yellow Cling Peaches packed in fruit juice, Minute Maid Orange Juice, Mott's Natural Style Applesauce, Mott's Apple Juice, Musselman Unsweetened Applesauce, Ocean Spray Grapefruit Juice, ReaLemon brand Natural Strength Lemon Juice from concentrate, Seneca Frozen Apple Juice, Sun Maid Natural Thompson Seedless Raisins, Sunsweet Prune Juice, Sunsweet Whole Prunes (these last three are high in calories), Treetop Apple Juice from Concentrate, Treetop Frozen Apple Juice Concentrate, Tropicana Orange Juice, Welch's Purple Grape Juice, and Welch's Red Grape Juice.

Baby Food: Beech-Nut Stage 1 Golden Delicious Applesauce, Gerber Strained Apple Juice, Gerber Strained Applesauce, Gerber Strained Mixed Fruit Juice, Gerber Strained Orange Juice.

When preparing food:

■ Keep fruit juice or cut fruit out of direct sunlight.

■ Do not leave fruit juice or cut fruit out of refrigerator for extended periods of time.

■ Prepare fruits immediately before they are to be cooked or served raw.

■ Prepare juices immediately before serving. When refrigerated and kept in a closed glass container overnight there is a little loss of

Vitamin C. (Note: The size of the container should be chosen so a minimum of air is left at the top.)
- Read labels carefully. Many canned fruits have extra sugar added. Select canned fruits packed in their own juice or water. If extra sugar (heavy syrup) has been added, drain off the liquid and wash the fruit.
- Buy citrus fruits in small quantities so they will be used promptly.

Dairy Products are important sources of protein, minerals, vitamins, and calcium. Milk products help rebuild tissue, maintain good bone strength, and provide for healthy teeth. When preparing dairy products, remember the following:

- Select fortified low-fat and skim-milk products. These contain fewer calories and less saturated fat and cholesterol. Fortunately they contain the same amounts of protein, minerals, and vitamins as those found in whole milk products.
- Cheeses, unfortunately, tend to be very high in cholesterol, very high in fat, and very high in salt.
- National brands of milk fortified with vitamins A and D are virtually the same.
- Preferable milk products and flavorings are: Carnation Evaporated Skim Milk, Carnation Instant Natural Malted Milk (218 mg. sodium), Carnation Instant Nonfat Dry Milk, Dannon Vanilla, Plain, Lemon Yogurt.
- Substitute nonfat dry milk, skim milk, or low-fat milk for whole milk in drinking and cooking. Make sure it's fortified with vitamins A and D. In most instances low-fat products are cheaper than whole milk. If you don't enjoy drinking skim milk (some children don't), try cooking with skim milk in soups, gravies, and puddings.
- Use yogurt as a substitute for sour cream.
- Substitute low-fat dairy dessert such as ice milk or frozen yogurt for whole-milk products. Be aware, however, that ice milk and fruit yogurt also contain sugar. As you can imagine, fruit-flavored yogurt has more sugar but plain yogurt usually is not favored by children. To get children to eat plain yogurt, add fresh fruit. NOTE: Children two and under should drink whole milk.

Protein Foods. Beef, fowl, and fish, selected vegetables and grains are important since they are rich in protein. Large amounts of the B vitamins are found in these foods as well. Meats build and repair body tissue—muscles, skin, hair, you name it. Meats are vital for healthy blood. Keep in mind the following when purchasing and preparing meat:

- USDA Prime: is higher in fat and calories and costs the most.
- USDA Choice: choice beef has a moderately high amount of fat, although less than USDA Prime.
- USDA Standard: some supermarkets feature a store brand of lean beef. USDA Standard is government inspected for wholesomeness. It has less fat than either choice or prime. Ground beef comes in different amounts of fat: regular is about 28 percent fat; lean is 23 percent; and extra lean is 18 percent.
- Beef and pork are higher in saturated fat and calories and are also more expensive than other kinds of protein.
- Select poultry and seafood to reduce the intake of saturated fat, cholesterol, and calories.
- Select water-packed tuna instead of tuna packed in oil.

These luncheon meats are low in sodium nitrate but high in sodium and fat:

- Buddig Smoked Sliced Beef
- Buddig Sliced Corned Beef
- Land O'Frost Beef
- Land O'Frost Chicken
- Oscar Meyer Olive Roll
- Mr. Turkey Cooked White Turkey Roll
- Mr. Turkey Golden No Salt Added Roast Turkey Breast
- Mr. Turkey Sliced Turkey Breast
- Bumble Bee Chunk Light Tuna in Water
- Bumble Bee Solid White Tuna in Water
- Chicken of the Sea Chunk Light Tuna in Water
- Star Kist Solid White Tuna in Water
- Chicken of the Sea Low-Sodium Chunk White Tuna in Water

These foods are relatively high in fat and sodium, with the exception of Mr. Turkey Golden No Salt Added Roast Turkey Breast and Chicken of the Sea Low-Sodium Chunk White Tuna in Water. Frozen fish, which are low in fat, cholesterol, and sodium:

- Gorton's Fishmarket Fresh Ocean Perch Filets
- Gorton's Fishmarket Fresh Sole Filets

Before cooking start thinking, and be sure to season meats without salt.

Breads, Cereals, and Grains. Whole-grain breads and cereals are important sources for carbohydrates, iron, and vitamins. Breads and cereals provide lots of energy, help in the formation of healthy blood, and provide resistance to disease. For maximum nutritional benefits, remember:

When preparing flour products, vegetable oil (corn, safflower, etc.) should be used in place of melted shortening when making pancakes, waffles, and other baked goods. Whole-grain flour may be used in rolls and bread recipes. Remember that whole-grain flour will not rise as high as regular white flour. You may wish to use half white flour and half whole grain.

When purchasing and preparing breads, consider the following:

- Purchase whole-grain bread made from stone-ground flour first.
- Next, purchase 100 percent whole-wheat or other grain bread. If you have time, check the ingredients. Milk and eggs increase the nutritive value of the bread. Both products, however, also increase the fat content.
- If you decide to purchase white bread, be certain that it is enriched.
- Dark bread means nothing. Most dark breads contain less or no whole grains—just molasses for coloring.
- The high-fiber breads are usually lower in calories.
- Whole-grain flour may be used in bread and roll recipes.

When purchasing cereals, consider the following:

- Whole-grain cereals are the most nutritious.
- Oatmeal (steel-cut or rolled oats)—the old-fashioned kind, not instant—is the best choice of cereals.
- The best "cold" cereals are Shredded Wheat and Cheerios (the latter is relatively high in salt).
- Puffed cereals are low in fat and salt.
- Granola contain nuts, seeds, raisins, and oats, but they are usually high in salt, fat, and sugar.

When purchasing rice and other grains, remember:

- Select whole-grain—brown—rice first. Parboiled or converted rice is a distant second. Instant and Minute rice are the lowest in nutrients.

Other grains include:

- Bulgur or burghul. Look for the irregular grains to see if the dark bran covering is still intact. If so, it has not been refined and has higher nutritive value.
- Buckwheat—although not really a grain, it is used as one. Buckwheat is usually eaten as flour or grits.

Pasta is made from a wheat called durum. Durum won't rise, so the durum wheat is refined into a white flour called semolina, which is mixed with water and other ingredients to make a dough and then shaped into spaghetti, macaroni, etc. This is a high-protein food and very nutritious. In some instances soy flour has replaced semolina or semolina is mixed with whole-wheat flours.

Vegetable Oils and Fats. As you read earlier, fats and oils can possibly play havoc with your heart and blood vessels. Consider the following when purchasing and selecting vegetable oils and fats.

Safflower and sunflower oils are the oils lowest in saturated fat. Soybean, corn, and olive oils are also relatively low in fat. Peanut oil and cottonseed oil tend to be higher, registering somewhere between 21 and 26 percent fat. Products such as coconut oil and palm oil should be avoided.

When it comes to fats, tub-type margarine and margarine stick types are best. Lard, beef tallow, and butter should be avoided. Some brand name margarines and oils which are relatively low in fat and have what scientists call a good P/S (polyunsaturated/saturated fats ratio) are:

Butter and Margarine:

- Hain Safflower Margarine
- Chiffon Soft Margarine—moderate sodium
- Fleischmann's Margarine—moderate amount of sodium
- Fleischmann's Stick Margarine—moderate amount of sodium
- Fleischmann's Unsalted Stick Margarine
- Mazola Margarine
- Mazola Diet Imitation Margarine
- Mazola Unsalted Margarine
- Mrs. Filbert's Family Spread
- Mrs. Filbert's Soft Corn Oil Margarine—moderate amount of sodium

Oil:

- Hollywood Safflower Oil
- Mazola Corn Oil
- Puritan Oil
- Sunlight Oil

Salad Dressings:

- Kraft Oil-Free Italian Dressings (as with all salad dressings, virtually no vitamins or minerals)
- Wishbone Liteline French Style Salad Dressing (still contains 60 percent of calories from fat)
- Wishbone Russian Salad Dressing (36 percent of calories from fat but high in sodium)

Again, beware of words such as "hardening," "saturated," "hydrogenation." These mean that perfectly good oils have been converted to bad oils.

Most reduced-calorie dressings are high in sodium. To make your own low-sodium dressing, mix ½ cup yogurt, ¼ cup vinegar, ¼ cup oil, 2 tbsp. Dijon mustard, ½ tsp. sugar with garlic and seasonings to taste. This is relatively low in fat and calories as well as sodium.

- If you like the flavor of butter when sautéeing, but wish to cut down on saturated fat, halve the amount of butter you normally use and substitute a good polyunsaturated vegetable oil such as a safflower oil for half of this reduced amount. If the food sticks to the pan, add a little water or broth.

Combination/Fabricated Foods. This group is a result and confirmation of the fact that we live in a nutritionally complex world. It includes most of those foods that come in a box, bag, jar, can, or from a fast-food restaurant. Most are combinations from several different food groups—for example, strawberry yogurt, cheeseburgers, macaroni and cheese, and so on. With these foods you need to look at the ingredients to determine their nutritional status.

One type of food in this group is fabricated foods—that is, those that come from the laboratory. Some examples include flavored gelatin, synthetic ice cream, soda pop, boxed dried potatoes, and synthetic eggs. These foods are marvels of technology, and they often contain added vitamins and minerals. But most have lots of sugar, salt, fat, and a mind-boggling array of unnecessary additives. I know that with kids it's often difficult to avoid these foods, so below I've listed some preferable (if you must) brand-name, high-tech foods:

The following contain relatively low amounts of fat (30 percent or less) but they are high in sodium:

- Armour Chicken Burgundy Classic Light Dinner
- Armour Seafood Natural Herbs Classic Light Dinner
- Armour Sliced Beef with Broccoli Classic Light Dinner
- Morton's Fried Chicken Dinner
- Morton's Veal Parmigiana Dinner
- Swanson Hungry-Man Turkey Dinner
- Swanson Turkey Dinner
- Stouffer's Glazed Chicken with Vegetable Rice Lean Cuisine

- Stouffer's Spaghetti with Beef Mushroom Sauce Lean Cuisine
- Swanson Hungry-Man Sliced Beef

The following foods have less than 100 milligrams of cholesterol per serving but they are high in sodium:

- Chef Boyardee Beef Ravioli in Tomato and Meat Sauce
- Franco-American Beef Ravioli in Meat Sauce
- Kraft Tangy Italian Sauce Spaghetti Dinner
- Old El Paso Refried Beans
- Chun King Beef Pepper Oriental Divider Pack
- Chun King Chicken Chow Mein Pouch

The following are pizzas that are relatively low in fat (30 percent or less) but they are high in sodium:

- Celantano Nine Slice Pizza
- Celantano Thick Crust Pizza
- Tree Tavern Frozen Cheese Pizza

Recommended soups:

- Campbell's Low-Sodium Chicken with Noodle Soup
- Campbell's Low-Sodium Tomato with Tomato Pieces—high sugar, however
- Progresso Minestrone Soup—moderate sodium

Sweets, Alcohol, and Other Beverages. These are the real nutritional bad guys. Sweets—foods that are high in sugar or corn syrup and often in fat as well—tend to be very low in nutrients. Nutritionists recommend that sweets should make up no more than 10 percent of the daily diet—about 240 calories a day; the average American eats about 500 calories of them a day. Recently sugar consumption has dropped considerably, but unfortunately this is little more than a shell game—food manufacturers have simply switched to corn sweeteners because they're cheaper. They're just as bad for you as sugar—in fact, they may even be worse, as corn has been linked to allergies in many people.

Finally in this category are beverages like soda pop, coffee, and tea. In general, their nutritive value is poor, although vitamin C has recently been added to some soft drinks. Those containing artificial sweeteners—saccharin and aspartame—are very popular. They seem to sidestep the most frequently voiced criticism of sweetened beverages—namely, that they provide empty calories. However, in this case the cure may be worse than the disease, as both saccharin and aspartame have problems of their own. Saccharin seems to increase the risk of cancer. In 1978 the National Academy of Sciences concluded that it's a weak carcinogen in animals and can probably cause cancer in humans as well. The National Cancer Institute has found that heavy saccharin users have a greater chance of developing bladder cancer (other experts, however, dispute these findings).

In 1981 the U.S. Food and Drug Administration approved the use of a new artificial sweetener, aspartame, and in 1983 it was approved for use in soft drinks. Although it's generally regarded as safe, some researchers are uncomfortable with its current widespread use. They fear that it may contribute to headaches or behavior changes in people who suffer from high blood pressure, Parkinson's disease, or insomnia. And of course, like saccharin, it panders to your sweet tooth.

Many sodas and other beverages also include relatively large amounts of caffeine—a stimulant that's entirely inappropriate for children. The typical American consumes about 1,250 milligrams of caffeine a day—five times the recommended maximum.

A Final Word: Salt and Additives. Although some salt is necessary in the diet, fresh unsalted foods contain plenty. Added salt admittedly enhances flavor, but try to keep its use to a minimum. The sodium that's contained in salt (as well as in monosodium glutamate, baking powder, and soy sauce) has been implicated as a major contributor to high blood pressure in those at risk from hypertension.

As for additives, they, too, are a mixed bag. More than 5,000 different kinds are used in food processing to preserve freshness and enhance the flavor of foods. Many of them have no adverse effects—yet, some are already known to be unhealthy. In general, try to avoid additives—especially the ones listed in Table 8-2.

TABLE 8-1 ■ *Nutrition Robbers*

ITEM	OTHER NAME(S)	WHERE USUALLY FOUND	POSSIBLE HEALTH PROBLEMS	NORMAL U.S. CONSUMPTION	RECOMMENDED U.S. CONSUMPTION	ALTERNATIV
Sugar	Sucrose, cane sugar, beet sugar, saccharose, corn syrup (sugar) starch, dextrose, corn sweetener	Cakes, cookies, pies, sweetened pop, fruit drinks, candy, cereals, canned fruit	Cavities, diabetes, hypoglycemia, hyperglycemia, heart disease, hyperactivity, gastrointestinal problems	500 cal. per day	200–250 cal. or 100 mg. per 1,000 cal.	Fruit
Fat	Lipid, triglyceride, diglyceride, monoglyceride	Animal products (beef, cheese, milk, pork, fish oils, butter), margarine, vegetable oils	Heart disease, cancer, possibly arthritis	(Cal. per day) Women: 1,000 Men: 1,260 Children: 1,000 42% of diet	(Cal. per day) Women: 720 Men: 900 Children: 720 30% of diet	Eat low-f meats an milk products. Use only polyunsa rated oils and margarin
Cholesterol		Organ meats, egg yolks, cheese, beef, pork, clams, chicken skin, whole milk	Heart disease	Adults: 600 mg. per day Children: 300 mg. per day	300 mg. or less per day or 100 mg. per 1,000 cal.	Limit int of fried meats an poultry t or 4 oz. p day (cook weight), 3 eggs pe week
Caffeine	Guaranine; methyltheo-bromine theine 1, 3, Q; 7-Tri-methy 1-2; 6-Dioxo-purine	Coffee, tea, chocolate bars and drinks, colas, cold remedies and stimulants, OTC analgesics	Heart and kidney disease, skipped heart-beats, cancer, gastric upset, anxiety, insomnia	1,000 mg. per day	No more than 300 mg. or 100 mg. per 100 lbs.	Limit co or cola to oz. a day

Salt	Sodium	Canned foods, bacon, bouillon cubes and powders, cheese, chili sauces, salad dressings, crackers, ham, luncheon meats, olives, butter, pickles, soy sauce, tenderizers	High blood pressure	8 to 15 grams	⅓ to 3 gm. per 100 mg.	

TABLE 8-2 ▪ *Additives*

AVOID	CAUTION
Artificial colorings: Blue No. 1, Blue No. 2, Citrus Red No. 2, Green No. 3, Red No. 40, Yellow No. 5	Artificial coloring Yellow No. 6
Aspartame	Artificial flavorings
Brominated vegetable oil (BVO)	Butylated hydroxyanisole (BHA)
Caffeine (for children and pregnant women)	Butylated hydroxytoluene (BHT)
Monosodium glutamate (MSG) (for children)	Caffeine (for nonpregnant adults)
Quinine	Carrageenan
Saccharin	Heptyl paraben
Sodium nitrate	Mono- and diglycerides
Sodium nitrite	Monosodium glutamate (MSG) (for adults)
	Phosphoric acid and phosphates
	Propyl gallate
	Sodium bisulfite
	Sulfur dioxide

CHAPTER **9**

Making Weight

The National Institute of Health has said that anyone who is 20 percent overweight, as determined by life insurance height/weight tables, suffers from the disease of obesity and requires medical help. It afflicts millions of children. Excess body fat strains the muscular and skeletal system as they work to support the additional load. It increases the heart rate and the work that the lungs must do. It makes exercise painful, thus promoting inactivity and an even greater propensity toward excess fat. It's a factor in high blood pressure, high cholesterol, diabetes, and some kinds of cancer. It can make surgery more of a risk. In addition, obesity can cause severe emotional and psychological damage, especially among children.

If your child's score on the skin-fold test was poor, fair, or average, he needs to reduce his proportion of body fat. This chapter offers a realistic weight-control plan to help him or her do that and some motivational tools to help keep your child (and you) on track.

Note those three key words: *realistic weight control*. Weight-loss plans—diets—are a dime a dozen. Many are useless or, worse, actually dangerous. Most are nutritionally unsound. Some may help you lose weight, but in most cases the dieter quickly regains the weight. Researchers tell us, in fact, that 95 percent of all diets fail.

A big part of the problem is that most diets try to achieve too much too soon. Quick weight loss is just about the worst way to achieve long-term weight control. The reasons are biological; sudden fasting signals the body's metabolism to slow down, thus burning even fewer calories. Thus, when the crash diet ends, pounds come back even more quickly than they came off—and usually a few extra ones come along too.

In addition, research has shown that "crash" dieting makes it even more difficult to lose pounds the next time you try to diet. It's as if the body's metabolism "learns" how to respond to cutbacks in food: the slowdown in metabolism occurs almost immediately, and despite the fasting, the pounds simply stay on.

There is a way out of this dilemma, but it's neither quick nor easy. Scientists have found time and again that gradual weight loss —no more than a pound or so a week—succeeds where crash diets fail. That means a much more difficult struggle for your child—as well as for you. Most of us can put up with almost anything for a week or two, but to stick with something over the course of months or years takes a profound commitment. You can expect plateaus and setbacks; you can expect your kids to "cheat" from time to time. But that's all part of the process, and as long as you strive toward a long-term goal, you can make it.

Obesity is simply a matter of arithmetic. As with any fuel, fat can be expressed in terms of energy (calories). A pound of fat is equivalent to 3,500 calories. So if your child's body burns 2,400 calories a day (which is about average) and consumes 2,500 calories a day, his body will be converting 100 calories a day into fat. In a month that will be close to a pound of fat. In a year it adds up to about ten pounds. The reverse is also true. If your child's body is burning 2,400 calories a day and he's eating only 2,300, he'll lose 100 calories of fat a day—or about ten pounds a year. (Note that the rate at which the body consumes calories can change in response to a number of things.)

As most of us know, losing weight doesn't always mean losing body fat. For one thing, a considerable amount of body weight is water. (Many crash diets achieve their spectacular first-week results through water loss, but such losses do nothing for long-term weight control. The weight starts returning as soon as the dieter drinks a glass of water.) You need to consider the proportion of body fat to lean tissue. You can diet for weeks, but if you lose body fat and lean tissue at equal rates, you'll be just as flabby (though smaller) when you're done.

The key to reducing body fat is to exercise while reducing the number of calories that are consumed. Exercise promotes the development of lean tissue (primarily muscle) at the expense of fat. After a few weeks of exercise your child may or may not weigh less (in fact, he may weigh more, since muscle weighs more than fat) but his body will be leaner. You'll be able to see the difference clearly. Exercise is also an important part of weight control (or, more accurately, fat control) because exercise—specifically the endurance type—speeds up the body's metabolism, making it easier to burn off excess calories.

HEALTHY-FOR-LIFE WEIGHT-CONTROL PROGRAM

This program will help your child lose fat, increase lean body tissue, and control his or her weight. Like the other Healthy-for-Life programs, it involves the entire family. There are four steps to the program:

Step 1: Be Positive

Step 2: Exercise Regularly

Step 3: Eat Right

Step 4: Be Assertive but Flexible

Step 1: Be Positive

A positive attitude may be the most important element of all in controlling weight. A "can-do" philosophy isn't easy to achieve,

■ ■ ■ ■ ■ ■ ■ ■ ■ ■ ■ ■

Adolescent Obesity

Obese teenagers will probably become obese adults. As a parent, you can do several things to help them control their weight.

1. Create a positive attitude about eating so that your children regard food as a friend that makes them healthy rather than a foe that makes them fat.

2. Create a positive mealtime environment that is relaxed and healthy.

3. Remove sugary and fatty snacks from your kitchen cupboard and refrigerator.

4. Encourage your teenager to get daily exercise—exercise along with him.

5. Avoid being critical. If you show too much concern, your teenager is probably going to be more resistant to losing weight. Keep your distance, but be supportive.

■ ■ ■ ■ ■ ■ ■ ■ ■ ■ ■ ■

though, especially if your child has heard a lot of negative talk about his weight at school or at home or if he's tried to lose weight before and failed. A study I conducted a few years ago showed that excess body fat is linked to low self-esteem. If your kids are overweight, I'm sure you're aware of how they suffer emotionally for it, so be sure that you present this weight-control program in a purely positive light. Emphasize that they need to lose weight so they'll be healthier, not because they're unattractive.

Don't let them think that they're failures or that they're being "punished" by the program. Also, give them an opportunity to express their anger and frustration. Praise them to the skies for every success, no matter how modest, and don't criticize them when they occasionally fall off the wagon—they probably feel worse about it than you ever will. In addition, don't dwell on the weight problem; help your child see that it's only a single part of his life and needn't color his entire perception of himself. Don't be afraid to seek some psychological counseling if it's needed; obesity is just as difficult to live with as any other chronic disease. Above all, teach your children to accept themselves for who they are, not how they look.

Step 2: Exercise Regularly

As discussed, exercise is a key element in a weight-control program. The exercise should be continual and rhythmic and should involve the entire body. Sports that require stopping and starting, such as bowling, golf, weight lifting, and softball, simply aren't effective in burning fat. That's not to say, of course, that your child shouldn't participate in such activities if he enjoys them. Just keep in mind that they aren't substitutes for the more active kinds of exercise that are necessary for weight control. (Table 9-1 gives you a rundown on the number of calories per minute that each consumes.) Here are some exercise suggestions, with pros and cons:

- Aerobic dancing is fun for all ages and both sexes. It's great if you like music and have a sense of rhythm, and when done properly it improves most components of physical fitness. On the down side, it's difficult to measure progress objectively, and the injury rate tends to be fairly high. Also, you may have some difficulty finding a program for kids, and a lot of "instructors" don't know what they're doing. Shop carefully!
- Bicycling and stationary bicycling are an excellent fat-control activity for kids. They provide a vigorous workout, strengthen leg muscles, and subject the body to very little wear and tear. How-

ever, many children pedal too slowly to derive the full fat-burning benefits. To burn fat have kids pedal fast, ride up hills, and use a gear that offers substantial resistance. Outdoor cycling can be dangerous, and should be done only with proper headgear and equipment; indoor cycling is safe, but kids find it boring.

- Cross-country skiing burns more calories than any other type of exercise. In addition, it's an excellent exercise for evaluating the success of a fitness program, since you can measure distance and speed. Obviously, the major drawback is the need for some snow. Also, a certain skill level is necessary to achieve full benefits; many beginners ski too slowly to burn significant numbers of calories. And, of course, the equipment can get expensive, and kids often find it a hassle to put on and take off the skis. Cross-country skiing usually works best as an occasional family activity.

- Indoor rowing and sculling stimulate the heart and lungs and the muscles of the upper and lower body. They also use a lot of calories. But sculling is expensive and seasonal, and it isn't appropriate for younger kids. Indoor rowing can be boring, and with a few exceptions (see Appendix D), most indoor machines don't do a good job of simulating real rowing.

- Running is an excellent way to reduce body fat. It conditions the legs and, like cross-country skiing, it permits you to measure progress by keeping track of distance and times. However, it isn't for everyone. It may shorten the muscles in the back of the leg, reduce flexibility, and make your child prone to injury and leg pain—especially if he's overweight. Also, while kids love to just run around in the yard, they're not so keen on logging miles. If parents run, they have a tendency to get their kids to run with them. That's fine, but recognize that they can get bored or may have trouble keeping up, so give them the opportunity to walk or skip as you run.

- Running in place and jumping rope are good rainy-day replacements for outdoor activities. Motivation can be a problem, as can measurement of progress. Also, both running in place and jumping rope can cause knee and ankle pain, though this problem is more prevalent in older people than in kids. Another problem with these activities is that as one becomes proficient, efficiency increases, thus the number of calories burned per minute drops

TABLE 9-1 ■ *Calories Burned per Minute During Aerobic Exercise*

	WEIGHT IN POUNDS												
	72–82	83–93	94–104	105–115	116–126	127–137	138–148	149–159	160–170	171–181	182–192	>193
AEROBIC DANCING												
Mild	2.8	3.1	3.3	3.4	3.8	4.1	4.3	4.6	4.8	5.1	5.3	5.6
Moderate	4.6	5.0	5.4	5.8	6.2	6.6	7.0	7.4	7.8	8.2	8.6	9.0
High	6.8	7.4	8.0	8.6	9.2	9.8	10.3	10.9	11.5	12.1	12.7	13.3
BICYCLING												
5.5 mph	2.5	2.5	2.9	3.2	3.4	3.6	3.8	4.1	4.3	4.5	4.7	4.9
10 mph	4.3	4.7	5.0	5.4	5.8	6.2	6.6	6.9	7.3	7.7	7.9	8.4
13 mph	6.8	7.4	8.0	8.6	9.2	9.8	10.3	10.9	11.5	12.1	12.7	13.0
CROSS-COUNTRY SKIING												
5 mph	7.3	7.9	8.5	9.2	9.8	10.4	11.0	11.7	12.3	12.9	13.3	14.2
9 mph	10.3	11.3	12.2	13.1	13.9	14.8	15.8	16.7	17.6	18.4	19.3	20.3
ROWING (strokes per minute)												
5	7.3	7.9	8.5	9.2	9.8	10.4	11.0	11.7	12.3	12.9	13.3	14.2
9	10.3	11.3	12.2	13.1	13.9	14.8	15.8	16.7	17.6	18.4	19.3	20.3

RUNNING

5.5 mph	6.8	7.4	8.0	8.6	9.2	9.8	10.3	10.9	11.5	12.1	12.7	13.3
6.0 mph	6.9	7.6	8.2	8.8	9.4	9.9	10.5	11.2	11.8	12.3	12.9	13.5
6.5 mph	7.1	7.8	8.3	8.9	9.5	10.2	10.8	11.4	12.0	12.6	13.2	13.8
7.0 mph	7.3	7.9	8.5	9.2	9.8	10.4	11.0	11.7	12.3	12.9	13.5	14.2
7.5 mph	7.8	8.5	9.1	9.8	10.4	11.2	11.8	12.5	13.2	13.8	14.5	15.2
8.0 mph	8.3	9.0	9.8	10.4	11.2	11.9	12.6	13.3	14.1	14.8	15.5	16.3

RUNNING IN PLACE/JUMPING ROPE (skips per minute or steps per minute—count left foot only)

50–60	5.3	5.8	6.3	6.7	7.2	7.6	8.1	8.5	9.0	9.4	9.9	10.3
70–80	5.8	6.3	6.8	7.3	7.8	8.3	8.8	9.3	9.8	10.3	10.8	11.3
90–100	6.8	7.4	8.0	8.6	9.2	9.8	10.3	10.9	11.5	12.1	12.7	13.3
110–120	9.3	10.2	10.9	11.8	12.6	13.4	14.2	15.0	15.8	16.7	17.4	18.3
130–140	12.4	13.5	14.6	15.7	16.8	17.8	18.9	20.0	21.1	22.2	23.3	24.3

SWIMMING (yards per minute)

20	3.1	3.4	3.7	3.9	4.2	4.5	4.8	5.0	5.3	5.6	5.8	6.1
30	4.3	4.8	5.1	5.5	5.8	6.3	6.7	7.0	7.4	7.8	8.0	8.5
35	5.6	6.1	6.6	7.1	7.6	8.0	8.5	9.0	9.5	10.0	10.5	10.9
40	6.3	6.8	7.3	7.8	8.3	8.9	9.4	10.0	10.5	11.1	11.6	12.2
45	7.2	7.8	8.3	9.0	9.6	10.3	10.8	11.5	12.1	12.8	13.3	13.9

FITNESS WALKING

3.5 mph	3.3	3.6	3.8	4.1	4.4	4.7	5.0	5.3	5.5	5.8	6.1	6.4
4 mph	3.6	3.9	4.3	4.5	4.8	5.2	5.5	5.8	6.1	6.4	6.8	7.0
4.5 mph	4.7	5.1	5.5	5.9	6.3	6.7	7.1	7.5	7.9	8.3	8.8	9.2
5 mph	5.8	6.3	6.8	7.3	7.8	8.3	8.8	9.3	9.8	10.3	10.8	11.3
5.5 mph	6.8	7.4	8.0	8.6	9.2	9.8	10.3	10.9	11.5	12.1	12.7	13.3

substantially. Of course jumping rope has long been a favorite activity of young girls. Encourage them in it.

■ Swimming is another possible exercise for weight loss. Since the water supports the body, injuries to the joints are virtually non-existent. In addition, progress is easily measured. However, you do need access to a pool, and your child must know how to swim. Unless the pool is enclosed, weather can be a factor. And as with the preceding exercises, efficiency may increase to the point where calories aren't being burned at a fast rate.

■ Fitness walking is good for just about everyone. It's easily worked into daily routines, the injury rate is low, and the entire family can do it together. What's more, it's fun—especially if it's scenic terrain (e.g., a nature walk). The major drawback is that improvement comes more slowly than with other fat-burning exercises. Often a family may wish to start out with a walking program and then graduate to more strenuous exercises.

For children age eight or older, have them choose one of the aerobic, fat-burning activities to do four times a week for 30 minutes (or an hour for fitness walking). If possible, have all family members participate. Use the following chart to record the calories expended:

My Personal Fat-Burning Activity Is _____.

	SUN.	MON.	TUES.	WED.	THURS.	FRI.	SAT.
WEEK 1							
WEEK 2							
WEEK 3							
WEEK 4							

Post this chart on the refrigerator door or bulletin board and use it as an incentive. For every 3,500 calories that are burned (one pound of body fat) give a small reward (for example, sweat bands, a T-shirt, or a health poster). Use a bigger health-related reward for every 35,000 calories—that is, 10 pounds—burned off (for example, running shoes or leg warmers). For 100,000 calories you can offer an even bigger reward, such as a new bicycle or all-weather running suit. (Make sure these rewards are for calories burned, not the amount of weight that's actually lost. By focusing on the first, you're rewarding behavior that's within the direct control of your child. That's vital to the success of the program.)

One extremely effective means of promoting physical activity is to permit your child to earn credit by burning "bonus" calories through a number of activities. None of them consume large amounts of calories, but they do add up. Also, they help focus your child's attention on his activity patterns. All of these "bonuses" involve doing things the "hard way"—that is, in ways that burn a few more calories. For example, sitting burns about two calories an hour more than lying down. That's not much, but if your child watches TV five hours a day, the difference adds up over time.

The list that follows offers some strategies for doing things the "hard way." Chart the results on the map on page 142 and provide some prearranged reward whenever your child reaches 3,500 calories. (Each square represents 10 calories.)

- Walk whenever you can. For every 100 to 120 steps, figure about four to five calories per minute.
- Climb trees, swing on swings, and play on seesaws at your playground—three to five calories per minute.
- Take the stairs rather than the elevator in apartment buildings or in stores. For every minute you walk the stairs, figure eight to ten calories.
- Every two hours get out of the chair at school or at home watching TV and move about for three to five minutes. Remember every 100 to 120 steps is worth four to five calories.
- Whenever you play sports try to play the most active position.
- Ride your bike as much as possible—five to seven calories per minute.

- After getting off the school bus make it a point to run home or to school—seven to ten calories per minute.
- If possible, walk to the store and help with the shopping—three to five calories per minute.
- When waiting for physical education to start, walk or run around the gym or playing field—four to ten calories per minute.
- During each commercial break get up and walk in place, run in place, do jumping jacks, bench step, jump rope, ride a stationary bicycle, or jump on a rebounder. Since a commercial lasts two minutes and in one hour there are at least six commercial breaks, your child would be getting about 12 minutes of exercise.
- For those not so vigorously inclined, try curl-ups, side leg raises, push-ups, curl-downs, wall push-aways, do some dumbbell curls, etc. These activities are worth an extra 20 to 50 calories if you do them for 12 minutes.
- Go sledding, skating, or skiing in the winter—four to ten calories per minute.

Other less ambitious ideas are:

- Never sit for more than an hour and a half at a time. Simply stand up.
- Never sit when you can stand, never stand when you can walk, never walk when you can run.
- Take the stairs when stairs and an escalator are side by side.

A couple of these activities can help burn off an extra 25 to 100 calories or more a day. That amounts to 2½ to 10 pounds of fat in a year.

Reproduce the following chart and record the number of calories your child uses "Doing Things the Hard Way."

Step 3: Eat Right

Keep a food diary. Nutritionists have a word for the current tendency to eat anywhere, anytime—"grazing." It's a dangerous habit and a major factor in obesity and other nutritional disorders. A first

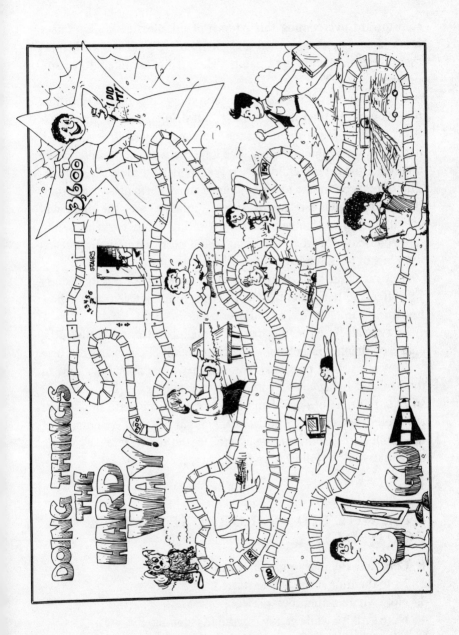

step toward overcoming this pattern of mindless eating is to keep track of it. For children ten and older, it's a good way of helping them focus on their eating habits. The results are likely to be surprising.

Encourage your kids to keep a food diary, recording everything that they put in their mouths: food, soft drinks, pencils, fingernails —everything. Have them include the time, place, associated feelings, and, if possible, calories. The food diary will show much more than what foods your child eats. It is also likely to show the relationship of his food intake to his emotional state. Particularly important is how food intake relates to stress. What's more, the diary will actually begin to change your child's eating habits by making him more conscious of what he's doing. He'll probably hesitate to reach for a bag of junk food and might choose the grapes instead.

As your child's eating program gets under way, the food diary will offer another benefit: It will permit him (and you) to see how his eating habits have changed over time.

You can also use the information in the food diary to start keeping charts of changes in behavior related to food. These charts can be a vivid way to show progress. You can chart just about any type of food-related behavior—for example, the number of between-meal snacks, the time of day when meals are eaten, or (with the help of the tables that show the nutritional content of food) the amount of fat, cholesterol, sodium, sugar, etc. in the diet. Here's a sample page that you can follow for a food diary:

INSTRUCTIONS FOR USING THE FOOD DIARY

1. Complete the diary right after eating.
2. Note the time when eating started.
3. Note where eating took place.
4. Note activity while eating (reading, watching TV, etc.)
5. Fill in the type of food and the amount.
6. If desired, look up and enter the number of calories in each food.

Food Diary

DAY: _____   DATE: _____

TIME	WHERE YOU WERE	ACTIVITY	YOUR FEELINGS	FOOD AND AMOUNT	CALORIES
6:00 A.M.–11:00 A.M.					
11:00 A.M.–4:00 P.M.					
4:00 P.M.–9:00 P.M.					
9:00 P.M.–6:00 A.M.					

Weight control for kids is an explosive issue. Some pediatricians are violently opposed to weight-control plans, saying that they can make kids obsessive about food or place them at risk for dietary deficiencies and poor growth patterns. However, it's equally true that fat children tend to have more heart-disease risk factors and are more likely to have weight problems as they grow up, and I'm convinced that you can get children to eat right and control calories without damaging their psyches or their bodies, Here's how:

Phase 1. Reduce or eliminate all the foods listed in the table below. (At the same time, of course, get them started on their fat-burning exercise program.) If your child is hungry, offer fresh vegetables, fruits, low-fat cheese, or milk products.

Monitor your children's weight. If it is dropping or staying the same and/or their body fat is decreasing after two months, stay with this plan. If not, have them move on to Phase 2.

TABLE 9-2 ■ *Phase 1 Eating Plan*

VEGE-TABLES	FRUIT	MILK AND MILK PRODUCTS	MEAT, FISH, LENTILS, NUTS, AND EGGS	GRAINS, BREADS, AND CEREALS	OILS AND FATS	SNACK FOODS AND OTHER
	Canned fruit in syrup, dried fruit, fruit "drinks"	Cream, ice cream, cream cheese, sour cream	Visible fat on any meat, bacon, corned beef, hot dogs, salami, luncheon meats, duck, goose, sausages, pâtés	Presweetened cereals	Lard, butter, margarine (ordinary)	Thick gravies, cake, pie, chocolate, cocoa, doughnuts, potato chips, pretzels, cookies, soda pop, coffee, candy

Phase 2. Eliminate *all* foods from the Phase 1 table, and now reduce or eliminate the following:

TABLE 9-3 ▪ *Phase 2 Eating Plan*

VEGE-TABLES	FRUIT	MILK AND MILK PRODUCTS	MEAT, FISH, LENTILS, NUTS, AND EGGS	GRAINS, BREADS, AND CEREALS	OILS AND FATS	SNACK FOODS AND OTHER
French fries, olives, pickles	Avocados and sweetened fruit	Cheeses (hard); blue, brick, camembert, cheddar; ice milk, processed cheese, whole milk, whole milk yogurt, puddings	Lean beef, lamb, pork, oily fish such as herring, mackerel, sardines, tuna in oil, deep-fried fish or poultry, spareribs, egg yolks, nuts, beans, peanut butter	Sweetened granola, packaged cereals with 10% or more sucrose, crackers, white bread, pasta	Mayonnaise, salad oils	Animal crackers, fig bars, popcorn with butter and salt, sherbet, jam, jelly, pizza, teas (other than herb)

Again, monitor your child's weight. If, after two months, your child has not lost weight or body fat, proceed to Phase 3.

Phase 3. Avoid foods from Phase 1, eat as little as possible from Phase 2 (preferably none), and cut the food from Phase 3 by one-fourth.

Monitor your child's progress. If his weight drops or stays the same and/or his body fat decreases, stay with this plan. If not, check with your pediatrician. Either your child is cheating or there is a metabolic problem of some kind.

TABLE 9-4 ■ *Phase 3 Eating Plan*

VEGE-TABLES	FRUIT	MILK AND MILK PRODUCTS	MEAT, FISH, LENTILS, NUTS, AND EGGS	GRAINS, BREADS, AND CEREALS	OILS AND FATS	SNACK FOODS AND OTHER
Canned vegetables, potatoes, canned salted vegetable juice, thick soups	Sweetened fruit juices	1 % to 2 % low-fat milk, cottage cheese	Shellfish (crab, shrimp), thick stews	Muffins	Special margarine	All snack foods

Step 4: Be Assertive But Flexible

Maintaining a weight-control program isn't easy, and friends and family can unwittingly make it even tougher. To be sure it's successful, you'll need to give your child some coaching on how to be assertive—how to say "no" firmly but gracefully to extra desserts, unhealthy behavior, and other obstacles.

Assertiveness is often confused with aggressiveness, but the two are quite different. An aggressive response is adversarial and confrontational; it tends to alienate. Assertiveness, by contrast, permits you to take a stand without embarrassing or angering the other person.

The only way I know for kids to master assertiveness is through practice and with lots of support and encouragement. Above all, keep the lines of communication open, so that your kids can discuss situations that come up and different ways in which they might have been handled.

When dealing with these sorts of issues keep the threshold concept in mind (page 38). In other words, set limits that permit some degree of failure. If your kid knuckles under to peer pressure and eats a burger, it's not the end of the world. Remind him that nobody bats a thousand, and encourage him to see the incident not as a failure but as something that can be improved upon in the future.

CHAPTER 10

How to Get Your Family to Eat Right

Eating behaviors are deeply ingrained, so you may have years of old habits to overcome. In addition, eating behaviors have a lot of emotional overtones. For better or worse, food is more than simply fuel for the body, it's a central part of many cultures. Likewise, eating isn't just a biological function, it's a profoundly social act as well, one of the ways we define who we are in relation to one another. If you refuse a second helping of Granny's secret-recipe potato salad—or, worse, pass it up altogether—you may find that you're no longer on speaking terms with her. If you don't feed your kids at least one serving of red meat a day, your Aunt Rose will swear they look sickly, no matter how fit they really are. Against this background you've got quite a job convincing your kids to forgo their after-school cheese doodles for a nice crisp apple. The only way you can get them to eat right is if you make a series of deliberate, well-thought-out changes.

Review your kids' scores on the Food Checkup. Chances are there are deficiencies in more than one area, but to succeed in changing behavior, you're better off selecting one area at first and concentrating on it—be it snacking, excessive sweets, a too-rich diet, picky eating, or junk food. With the help of the Food Checkup, you probably won't have too much difficulty choosing the area that's most in need of attention in your family. Once you do, simply turn to the corresponding section in this chapter and follow the suggestions you find there.

TOO MANY SNACKS

Children have powerful role models for snacking: Three-quarters of adult Americans have bedtime snacks. Morning and afternoon coffee breaks are an American institution, and have even been negotiated into most labor contracts, so it's no wonder that by age 13 the typical American child gets a fourth of his daily calories from snacking.

I'm convinced that once children get into the habit of snacking, it's almost impossible to stop; if you try, be prepared to put up with a hungry kid pestering you for food all the time. What, then, can you do? Surrender gracefully; learn to live with snacks, but make them nutritious. Here's a five-week plan for transforming junk-food snacks into healthy snacks:

Week One

- Try not to buy candy, crackers, cookies, etc. "just to have in the house in case someone drops in." You must learn to be truthful if you are going to be successful.
- If you must have these foods, place them out of reach, out of sight, and out of mind.
- In place of these traditional snacks, make the following readily available after school:
  a) fresh fruit, or canned in water or its own juice
  b) cheese; if your kids demand crackers, buy the low-salt kind
  c) yogurt
  d) half sandwich (whole grain, of course)
  e) fruit juice
  f) cereal with milk

g) whole-grain muffins
h) raw vegetables

Week Two

- Continue all points of Week One, but limit snack time. Example: No snacks after 4:00 or approximately an hour and a half before mealtime. Snack in the evening two hours *after* a meal.

Week Three

- Do Weeks One and Two, but also prepare school snacks as outlined in Week One.
- Prepare the following snacks for after school:
  a) unsalted nuts
  b) popcorn (unsalted or lightly salted, no butter, special margarine okay)
  c) cut up raw vegetables in plastic containers or plastic bags
  d) dried fruit

Week Four

- Do Weeks One through Three. Avoid doing several things at snack time. No reading, watching TV, or talking on the phone. When you snack, snack.

Week Five

Things should be running more smoothly by now. Hang tough. You will lose some battles, but your goal is to win the war.

- You and your child can keep a snacking diary. Keep it simple, by simply making check marks. Place on the refrigerator door.

Snack Record

	MORNING	AFTERNOON	EVENING
Vegetables			
Fruit			
Milk/Dairy			
Protein Foods			
Grains			
Crackers			
Cookies			
Pies			
Fruit Drinks			
Ade Drinks			
Soda Pop			

REDUCING FAT AND CHOLESTEROL

Reducing the intake of fatty foods is a cornerstone of a healthy diet. Unfortunately, fat isn't always an obvious bad guy like sugar—many seemingly healthy foods are loaded with fat. In fact, rich food, such as heavy cream sauces and well-marbled steaks, are often thought of as "premium" foods—the best of the best—so eliminating excess fat may take some rethinking on your part about what constitutes good food. Here's a six-month plan for reducing fats in your family's diet:

Month One

- When purchasing meat select lean, well-trimmed cuts of beef or pork.

Ranking of oils/margarines (generic)

Best (Use at will)
- Safflower Oil
- Sunflower Oil
- Corn Oil
- Tub Margarine (liquid safflower)
- Soybean Oil

Good (Use frequently)
- Sesame Oil
- Soybean Oil (lightly hydrogenated)
- Tub Margarine (liquid corn oil)

Fair (Use sparingly)
- Cottonseed Oil
- Imitation (diet margarine)
- Peanut Oil
- Stick or Tub Margarine
  (partially hydrogenated/hardened)
- Stick Margarine (liquid corn oil)
- Vegetable Shortening (hydrogenated)
- Mayonnaise

Poor (Avoid)
- Olive Oil
- Lard
- Palm Oil
- Coconut Oil
- Butter

▪ When cooking use vegetable oil (preferably non-hardened or -hydrogenated) or special soft margarine in place of butter, shortening, or lard. (See box, page 156.)
▪ Replace two red-meat meals each week with poultry or fish.

Month Two

▪ Continue Month One recommendations.
▪ Switch from whole milk to 2 percent fat milk products.
▪ Cut in half your consumption of high-fat foods such as bacon, cream, cold cuts, cakes, pie, cookies, ice cream, and other rich, creamy desserts.
▪ Eat two fewer egg yolks each week.

Month Three

▪ Continue previous two months' efforts.
▪ Avoid nondairy creamers.
▪ Limit the number of organ-meat meals you have each week to two.
▪ Cut in half the amount of cream cheese or cheddar cheese you have each week.

Month Four

▪ Continue previous three months' efforts.
▪ Whenever recipe calls for two eggs use two egg whites and only one yolk.
▪ Limit intake of meat, fish, poultry to eight ounces (cooked weight) per day.
▪ When ordering salad in restaurants ask for the dressing on the side. Use sparingly. Make homemade salad dressings from safflower, corn, or sunflower oil.

Month Five

- Switch from 2 percent fat milk products to 1 percent—skim milk if possible.
- Limit fried foods to one serving per week.
- Limit cheeses to low-fat variety. No more than two servings of high-fat cheeses per week.
- Cut in half again the number of high-fat foods you eat—bacon, cream, cold cuts, and rich desserts.

Month Six

- Replace five red-meat meals each week with poultry, fish, or high-protein vegetables.
- Eat no more than three egg yolks a week.
- Limit the number of meals you have every two weeks that have organ meats as a base to one.
- Limit your intake of meat, fish, and poultry to four ounces (cooked weight) per day.
- Prepare and eat poultry without skin.

THE PICKY EATER

Picky eaters are the bane of early parenthood. However, remember to keep picky eating in perspective. As long as your child is eating a reasonably balanced diet and his doctor isn't concerned about his growth rate, it doesn't really matter if he doesn't clean his plate at dinnertime. In fact, he may grow up healthier and live longer than so-called good eaters. Studies have shown, for example, that mice who are a little thin and underfed live significantly longer than their plump counterparts.

So, with that thought in mind, I offer you my not-quite-foolproof recommendations for winning over the picky eater:

With very young children, try arranging the food in the shape of a face or animal. (If they still don't eat it, at least you can sign it and hang it on the refrigerator.)

If your child won't drink milk. For some reason, parents panic if their kids don't drink milk. Maybe it was all that public relations over the years from the milk-marketing people, who touted milk as "nature's most perfect food." In reality, milk is rather high in fat, and it lacks some important nutrients. In addition, many people have milk allergies that can result in permanent intestinal damage if they drink too much milk.

These objections notwithstanding, milk actually is a good source of nutrition—especially for girls, who require plenty of calcium to help prevent osteoporosis (thinning of the bones) later in life. But if your kids don't like to drink milk, there are other milk products that will do just as well. (Incidentally, I don't recommend adding chocolate or other flavors to the milk to get kids to drink it. These flavorings are usually high in sugar and fat—usually coconut fat.)

As an alternative to milk, try substituting milk products such as yogurt—with or without fruit or flavoring. Cheese (avoid those with the word "processed" on the label) is also good; many kids like cottage cheese covered with fruit. Ice milk once a week is okay. Also you can sneak milk (liquid or powdered) into other foods that your child does eat, such as bread, casseroles, hot cereals, puddings, soups, and pancakes. And for some reason it seems that kids who hate milk in a glass will accept it poured over their cereal.

Many kids enjoy mixing milk (preferably low-fat) with fruit in a blender; a little sugar or honey may reduce the tartness.

Your Child Refuses to Eat Vegetables. Children refusing to eat veggies isn't uncommon. (Of course there are exceptions.) To get your kids to eat them, do the following:

1. Use fresh vegetables whenever possible. Be sure to keep them crisp—do *not* overcook.
2. Buy a steamer to fit inside your pans so vegetables won't sit in the water when cooking.
3. In the beginning top vegetables with your children's favorite

▪ ▪ ▪ ▪ ▪ ▪ ▪ ▪ ▪ ▪ ▪ ▪ ▪

Picky Eaters

Evette M. Hackman, Ph.D., R.D., provides some cogent advice for "picky" eaters.

▪

Make eating at table comfortable.

▪

Use child-size utensils.

▪

Use cups that are spill-proof.

▪

Use plates with a rim to help serve as a stopper when trying to scoop up food with a spoon.

▪

Offer a wide range of wholesome food.

▪

Recognize that kids will eat less on some days.

▪

Keep portions small.

▪ ▪ ▪ ▪ ▪ ▪ ▪ ▪ ▪ ▪ ▪ ▪ ▪

melted cheese, then graduate to using soft tub margarine instead of cheese. In time gradually cut back on the cheeses and margarines until you use a very small amount.

4. "Doctor" vegetables with soups—top green beans with mushroom soup and onions.

5. Try fresh vegetables with dips. While dips may not be as healthy, they can get children to eat vegetables. Try kohlrabi, carrots, radishes, turnips, broccoli, and cauliflower.

6. Be cautious with vegetables such as cabbage, sweet potatoes,

zucchini, pumpkin, and beans (lima, kidney, green). Camouflage them by combining them in recipes. Use cabbage in cole slaw; sweet potatoes, zucchini, pumpkin in breads or puddings; beans in casseroles, soups, or three-bean salad.

7. Combine vegetables. With frozen vegetables, take a little from several bags and cook together.
8. Try oriental-style frozen vegetables.
9. Be cautious with salt. If a recipe calls for salt, don't use it, or cut the amount in half. The family can season to taste at the table. But be cautious—they may oversalt. The best strategy is to add one half the amount called for in recipes, then one-third, then one-fourth. Most families tolerate those gradual reductions.

BEATING THE JUNK-FOOD BLITZ

I'm convinced that an addiction to junk food is simply the result of another, more powerful addiction—the addiction to television. It's not just the sedentary nature of TV viewing. The typical American child is bombarded every year with hours upon hours of sugary food commercials. Through television your kids receive the equivalent of 13 to 14 sales pitches a day for junk food. Against such an onslaught, whole-wheat bread and fresh vegetables scarcely stand a chance.

Before you can wean your kids off these foods, you will need to start an ad campaign yourself. Try following this six-month plan:

Month One

- Limit TV viewing. Difficult at best, but this approach reduces the exposure of your children to TV's advertising messages.
- Make your kids consumer conscious. When you watch TV with your child start a rating game: On a scale of 1 to 10 how does the

add stack up—appealing . . . innovative . . . whatever? Then
follow with the biggie: What are they really selling, the "sizzle"
or the steak? Kids really enjoy unmasking TV advertisers.

- Point out flaws in advertising. A cereal might be loaded with
essential vitamins, but it is also filled with sugar, which rots your
teeth. Tell your children that.

Month Two

- Purchase low-salt crackers, chips, and pretzels.
- Cut in half the amount of cola beverages your child drinks each
week.
- Cut in half the amount of milk chocolate your child eats each
week.

Month Three

- Cut in half the amount of ade-type drinks your child has each
week.
- Select granola bars that are low-fat, -salt, and -sugar.
- Have your child eat no more than three meals a week at a fast-
food-type restaurant. When you do eat at one order fruit juice
instead of shakes or soda pop beverages. Select 2 percent butterfat
(or less) milk instead of whole milk.
- Have your child select fish sandwiches over burgers to keep fat
content lower; salt content will be about the same.

Month Four

- Have your child eat no more than two meals a week at fast-food-
type restaurants. Also select fries without salt, select from salad
bar, or pick a restaurant that provides potatoes, tacos, or pizza
versus burgers.

Month Five

- Cut in half the number of meals you prepare that come in a box or a bag. That is, use caution with TV dinners, meat or fruit pies, luncheon meats.
- Select packaged cereals that are low in salt and sugar.

Month Six

- Have your child avoid fast-food restaurants that do not have salad bars. Attempt to get half of the calories from these restaurants from the salad bar. Or select a plain hamburger instead of one with all the trimmings. Learn to put on your own lettuce, tomatoes, etc. from the salad bar on the hamburger minus the sauces.
- If for some reason you or your child positively cannot avoid a hamburger with the trimmings, round out the rest of your meals for the day with low-calorie foods such as vegetables, fruit, and whole-grain breads.

The following table summarizes the personal eating plan all family members should strive to achieve. This plan ensures low-sugar, -cholesterol, -salt, -fat, -alcohol, and -caffeine eating and drinking. Post it on your refrigerator or bulletin board.

TABLE 10-1 ■ *Personal Eating Plan*

COLUMN 1	COLUMN 2	COLUMN 3	COLUMN 4
High Fat, Cholesterol, Salt, Sugar, and/or Low Fiber ■ One serving or less a month	Moderately High Fat, Cholesterol, Salt, Sugar, and/or Low Fiber ■ One serving or less a week	Moderately Low Fat, Moderate Cholesterol, Salt, Sugar, and Fiber ■ Two to three servings a week	Low Fat, Cholesterol, Salt, Sugar, and/or High Fiber ■ Daily

(continued on next page)

FOOD GROUPS

	COLUMN 1	COLUMN 2	COLUMN 3	COLUMN 4
Group 1 Nonstarchy Vegetables and Starchy Vegetables	Fried vegetables (e.g., onion rings), okra, pickles, chips, french fries, or olives	Canned vegetables, fresh or frozen vegetables prepared in butter, cream, or sauce. Canned vegetables, tomato juice, sauerkraut, or cole slaw	Fresh or frozen vegetables, margarine added, or low-salt canned vegetables	Fresh or frozen vegetables, slightly cooked or steamed
Group 2 Fruit	Fruit Roll-Ups or fruit "drinks"	Sweetened or fruit in heavy syrup, or avocado	Fruit juice with sugar added by food-processing company	Fresh raw fruit, "no-sugar-added" fruit juices
Group 3 Milk and Milk Products	Cream, cheese, half-and-half, or ice cream	Whole milk, cheeses, yogurt, cottage cheese, fruit yogurt, frozen yogurt, buttermilk, puddings, ice milk, sour cream	2 % fat milk, cheese, yogurt, cottage cheese, fruit yogurt, frozen yogurt, buttermilk, or puddings with skim milk	Low-fat (1%) or less milk, cheeses, plain yogurt, or cottage cheese
Group 4 Protein Foods	Organ meats, bacon, frankfurters, salt pork, fatty fish (sardines, mackerel, fish eggs), luncheon meats, ham, salted nuts and seeds	Duck, goose, or vegetable protein meats such as meatless bacon	Lean beef, egg yolks, tuna in oil, veal, shellfish, peanut butter, unsalted nuts or seeds	Poultry (no skin), fish, egg white, tuna in water (watch salt), dried beans, lentils, peas, split peas, tofu

Group 5 Breads and Cereals	Presweetened cereals, crackers, or pretzels	Low-salt crackers, granolas, biscuits, white bread, or granola bars	No-coconut palm-oil granolas, refined cereals, pasta (refined), white rice, pasta (spaghetti, macaroni)	Whole-grain breads and cereals, shredded wheat, brown rice, bran, wheat germ, whole-grain pasta (spaghetti, macaroni)
Group 6 Fats and Oils	Butter, coconut, cream gravy, shortenings, or lard	Salad dressings, tartar sauce, diet margarines, hydrogenated or hardened oils	Special margarine or mayonnaise	Special soft tub margarines, vegetables oils (corn, safflower)

In Columns 1 to 3, a listing refers to one serving. For example, in Column 2 you may have one serving from that food group only.

Table 10-2 gives you similar guidelines on combination foods, sweets, and beverages.

TABLE 10-2 ▪ *Combination Foods, Sweets, and Beverages*

	COLUMN 1	*COLUMN 2*	*COLUMN 3*	*COLUMN 4*
FOODS	One serving or less a month	One serving or less a week	Two to three servings a week	Anytime
Group 7 Combination Foods	TV dinner, dehydrated soups, combined soups	Hamburger, cheeseburger	Cheese pizza, meat loaf, regular spaghetti, macaroni and cheese, Swiss steak, beef/cheese taco, chow-mein chicken, low-salt soy sauce	Stew, chili, whole-grain spaghetti, bean/cheese taco, tuna/noodle casserole, lentil/rice casserole, homemade soups

(continued on next page)

	COLUMN 1	COLUMN 2	COLUMN 3	COLUMN 4
FOODS	One serving or less a month	One serving or less a week	Two to three servings a week	Anytime
Group 8 Sweets and Beverages	One serving alcohol exceeding 12%, regular cake, cupcakes, cookies or pies, ice cream, doughnuts	One serving 12% or less alcohol, angelfood cake, jams, jellies, hard candy, Fudgecicles or Popsicles, carbonated beverages (sweetened or nonsweetened), syrup, molasses, colas	Tea, coffee	Decaffeinated coffee, tea, mineral water

▪   ▪   ▪   ▪   ▪   ▪   ▪   ▪   ▪   ▪   ▪   ▪

Fast-Food Blues

Here is some help if your child eats frequently at fast-food restaurants.

1. Look for fast-food restaurants with salad bars. Wendy's, Burger King, Sizzler, Carl's Jr., and many pizza places have salad bars.
2. Roast beef sandwiches have less fat than hamburger. Winners include Roy Rogers Roast Beef, Arby's Roast Beef, Hardy's Roast Beef, and D'Lite Burgers.
3. Order the smallest, plainest hamburger.

According to Evette Hackman, Ph.D., R.D., Consulting Nutritionist at the Stevens Health Clinic in Edmonds, Washington, here are items to choose at fast-food restaurants.

- A & W: grilled chicken, lettuce, tomato on wheat bun.
- Arby's: turkey sandwich, with lettuce and tomato (adapted from Turkey Deluxe), junior roast beef, plain baked potato, vanilla or chocolate shake to share.
- Burger King: salad bar, fresh fruit, small hamburger, orange juice, milk.
- Carl's Jr.: salad bar, fresh fruit, Happy Star burger, California roast beef sandwich, orange juice, milk, hot chocolate, plain baked potato, English muffin, slice of Swiss cheese.
- Church's Fried Chicken: corn on the cob; emergency option—take the skin off the chicken.
- Domino's Pizza: cheese pizza, cheese pizza with veggies.

Continued

- Jack In The Box: Club Pita. Avoid the large chef salad, taco salad, and pasta and seafood salad, they're loaded with fat.
- Kentucky Fried Chicken: corn on the cob, mashed potatoes; emergency option—take the skin off the chicken.
- McDonald's: English muffin, prepackaged salads, ice-cream sundae with sauce but no whipped cream.
- Wendy's: baked potato, chili, chicken sandwich on multigrain bun.
- Mexican food: soft tortillas (unfried) with beans, small amounts of cheese, chicken, lettuce, and tomatoes. Avoid guacamole, sour cream, tostadas, tacos, or other crisp, fried tortillas.

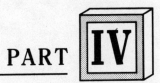

PART **IV**

Where Do We Go From Here?

CHAPTER 11

The Bad Side of the Good Life

O f all our modern-day blessings, two in particular have contrib-
uted to our children's physical decline. The average American
child watches between three and seven hours of TV a day and rides
twenty-two miles a day in a car, bus, or other form of motorized
transportation. As a result kids are sitting down for a minimum of
three and a half hours a day every day of the year. On school days
they get another six and a half hours of sitting. Add an hour of
sitting for meals, nine to ten hours for sleeping, an hour for getting
dressed and talking with friends (a conservative estimate if my
house is any gauge), and you've accounted for most of the day.

To determine just how active children are, I conducted a study
of 450 children. I had 36 children in the study wear something
called a Holter monitor—a device that looks something like a Sony
Walkman and records its wearer's heart rate throughout the day.

The study used heart rate as a barometer of each child's activity
—the greater the activity level, the higher the heart rate. For example, a child's heart rate when he sleeps may be 90 to 100 beats
per minute (bpm). In the classroom it may be 100 to 130; when the
child runs it may rise to 160 or more. Here are the results. I think
you'll be as shocked as I was.

Kids have not always been sedentary. In the forties and fifties

TABLE 11-1 ▪ *Average Heart Rates of Children Throughout a*
Day

HEART-RATE RANGE	ACTIVITY LEVEL	HOURS, MINUTES	PERCENTAGE OF 24 HOURS
Less than 129 bpm	Sedentary or mild	23 hrs., 3 min.	96%
130–159 bpm*	Moderate	43 min.	3%
160 and over*	Vigorous	14 min.	1%

* Heart rates may have been higher at times due to the fact that they were playing video games, anxious about a test, or experiencing peer conflict.

** Since the children usually went to bed or sat watching TV right after taking the Holter device off, we assumed that their heart rates were at 100 beats per minute or less during sleep.

kids had greater opportunities for outdoor play (what else could they do after school?). Children in the sixties had TVs, but still a good bit of outdoor activity. But most of the children of the seventies and the eighties are captivated by television and video games. Saturday mornings are usually spent watching cartoons.

Research shows a consistent decline in physical activity. In 1967 researchers found that European children aged 13 to 15 spent 1.2 hours a day either walking, playing sports games, or riding bicycles, and three-quarters of an hour running and engaging in other vigorous activities. By contrast, researchers doing studies in Europe and elsewhere today support our findings that children spend only three-quarters of an hour on moderate exercise and one-quarter of an hour on vigorous activity. Furthermore, the rash of child molestations, kidnappings, and murders has created a paranoia that has caused parents to keep their children close to home. As a consequence children's normal activity patterns are greatly restrained. Outside of school kids don't get decent exercise. Many urban children live in apartments. Their playgrounds are the streets and sidewalks—less than desirable places to become fit. The parks, Y's, and clubs are rapidly becoming a thing of the past and too expensive.

Moreover, less and less money is available for state and local recreation programs. One major U.S. city fired one-third of its recreation staffers. According to the San Diego City Recreation Department, in 1978 the city of San Diego had after-school recreation leaders at 97 elementary schools. Today they have none! Some cities are now forced to charge for services in providing basketball and softball leagues to help make ends meet.

Clearly the child who comes from an urban neighborhood—especially a less affluent one—is getting shortchanged when it comes to physical activity. But things are not much better down on the farm. Studies in Canada and Czechoslovakia suggest that today's urban children are more fit than rural children. The reasons for this surprising result are that the rural children have even more limited opportunities for organized sports and don't walk as far to school (1.2 kilometers rural versus 2.4 kilometers urban) because a bus picks the rural children up close to home.

Unfortunately, physical education has recently sputtered in schools. Budget cuts and the drive back to the three R's have made exercise an unaffordable luxury for some people. If educational cuts must be made, physical education is usually the first. Additionally, while the quality of education has been a political issue, government officials have not seemed concerned about the quality of *physical* education that their children are receiving.

In the past few years, for example, elementary schools have greatly curtailed physical education instruction. In California three-quarters of all schools studied have terminated or reassigned physical education teachers since 1977. Consequently, the classroom teachers have been forced to pick up the slack. A growing number of high schools have made physical education optional. The rationale is that the kids will be free, then, to do "their own thing" and teachers will be forced to be innovative and offer exciting courses. Unfortunately, less than 50 percent of the children participate in optional physical education curricula.

On the average, children of fifth grade and above in the United States spend only 3 percent of their school day in physical education or physical activity. By contrast, in Japan 18 percent of the children's day is spent in physical activity. This figure is even more striking when you realize that school in Japan runs from 8:00 A.M. to 3:30 or 4:00 P.M., Monday through Friday, and 8:00 A.M. to 12:00 noon on Saturday. Too, children go to school year-round, with only a two- or three-week break in March and August and a one-week pause at the New Year.

For some unexplainable reason there has also been the tendency for some physical education teachers simply to "roll out the ball." That is, they do not provide basic instruction. Many physical education programs do not emphasize the most basic motor skills of running, jumping, throwing, catching, skipping, hopping, and swimming. On the plus side for physical educators, however, the 1987 National Children and Youth Fitness Study II showed that youngsters who performed better on cardiovascular fitness tests were children who received instructions from a physical education specialist.

Furthermore, we have our priorities backward with respect to physical activity and food. If a team wins a game, we take them out to eat. If they lose a game, we tell them to take laps and do push-ups—"Gotta toughen these kids up. Make 'em winners." Children learn very quickly that if they drop a ball, miss a tackle, or make a poor play, they will be told to take laps or do extra push-ups. If they win a key game, strike out the opposing batter, or hit a home run, they will be taken out to eat. The result is obvious. Children view food as a reward, physical activity as punishment.

Unfortunately, parents aren't hot and bothered by this punishment approach. A National Youth Sports Research and Development Survey conducted in 1988 found that 60 percent of the parents think that extra exercise, such as running laps, is acceptable discipline in sports programs. Fred Negh, President of the National Youth Sports Coaches Association, hits the nail on the head about this attitude by saying, "Doing laps [as punishment] turns into a sour attitude toward exercise later in life."

Closely allied is the fact that team sports such as basketball, softball, and football have very little long-term benefits. Kids get more benefit from individual achievement sports such as swimming, running, and other lifetime sports. Of course team sports do have value —they teach team play, the necessity of cooperation, rules of the game. But these activities should not be considered physical fitness activities. They are activities a child can enjoy *after* he or she is fit.

FIT FOR SPORTS

As parents, we tend to assume that if our children participate in sports, they are fit. Unhappily, this is not always the case. Participation in organized sports often triggers an increased interest in fitness (tests show most athletes don't play a sport to get into shape, but get in shape so they can better play their sport), but the fact that your child is on the team doesn't ensure that he or she is getting enough exercise. For example, tests done on professional baseball players at the end of the season (who don't engage in rigorous training programs during the season) show that they are in no better shape than the average American. On the other hand, similar tests done on marathon runners or swimmers would likely indicate that such athletes are in top physical condition. It all depends upon the sport.

Participation in organized sports, however, generally creates a cycle—the more your children participate, the more fit they will want to become so they can excel at their sport. Proper warm-up and conditioning exercises also enhance fitness.

Help your children get the most out of organized sports by following these tips:

■ Make sure your child competes against opponents of similar athletic ability. A child who competes against a far superior opponent will tire quickly and become frustrated. By the same token, if an opponent is much less athletic, the child won't get a workout at all and will probably become bored.
■ Make sure your child is actually participating as a team member. Standing in right field or on the sidelines won't provide much of a workout. In that case, provide supplemental exercise.

- ■ Check out the sports program. Before enrolling your child in Little League or other organized sports programs, talk to the coach. Is his or her goal to make sure each child participates or is the coach more interested in winning a championship? If the latter is the case, and your child is still a rookie, chances are he or she will spend most of the time on the bench. Your child may get a better workout and feel more like a champ on another team or in another league.
- ■ Finally, don't get too involved and lose sight of the program's purpose—your children having fun and, hopefully, some healthy exercise.

The good news about sports programs, as highlighted by the National Children and Youth Fitness Study, is that children participating in community-based physical education programs tend to have better cardiovascular endurance and lower body fat.

CHAPTER 12

What to Look for in Physical Education

Physical education classes, extracurricular programs at Y's and recreation centers, and organized team sports such as Little League have a tremendous potential for helping your children become fit. But they don't always live up to that potential. All too often they're actually counterproductive—one lousy coach can turn your kids off to physical fitness.

"Those who can, do. Those who can't, teach. Those who can't teach, teach gym." Sadly, that old joke speaks volumes about the value we place on physical education in our culture. For far too long it's been a stepchild to educators and policymakers, seen as little more than a social-welfare program for college athletes who weren't good enough to make the big leagues. There are many good coaches and physical education teachers in our schools, but there are also far too many who don't know—or don't care—enough about what they're doing.

A large part of the problem comes from a tendency to confuse athletics programs with physical education. If a school has a winning football team, the coaches and phys ed teachers are community heroes and nobody questions whether the physical education program is any good. But be suspicious of a school with winning varsity teams—it suggests that the coaches are focusing most of their efforts on programs that benefit perhaps 5 percent of the school students.

One reason that physical education programs tend to stress athletics is that most of the instructors are or have been athletes themselves. Not surprisingly, those who major in physical education in college are usually those who tend to be "good at sports"—in fact, most are college athletes. And at the college level the phys ed professors are almost exclusively former athletes. Athletes teaching athletes—it's a closed system.

There are, fortunately, ways you can improve your child's school wellness and fitness programs. Don't by shy and do exercise your authority. When parents complain the great majority of superintendents will immediately call the department in question and find out what is going on. As a parent, however, you should get your facts straight. Make sure you have done your homework. (You may be pleasantly surprised that the school is providing excellent health/physical education programs and a good school health environment.) Furthermore, there is strength in numbers. Get other parents to cooperate with you. You'll be amazed at what you can accomplish if you are committed, united, forthright, caring, and well prepared.

Every child should benefit from the school's physical education program. The value of exercise in the school curriculum is obvious. Parents have a right to demand quality education, and a critical component is a physical education curriculum that is contemporary and meets the needs of the children.

To help you determine if your schools are providing physical education programs most beneficial to your children, use the following grading system.

Level of Participation

Low		High	
1	2	3	1. Does your school provide at least one period per day of vigorous (heart rates above 160 beats per minute) physical activity?
1	2	3	2. Does your school offer instruction in lifetime activities such as walking, running, swimming, bicycling, aerobic dancing, tennis, badminton, and skiing?
1	2	3	3. Does your school provide tests to determine children who are unfit—that is, lack flexibility, strength, and cardiovascular endurance?
1	2	3	4. Does your school provide physical activity opportunities for children who are obese, unfit, and unskilled?
1	2	3	5. Does your school provide physical education programs for children with special problems such as the retarded and the handicapped?
1	2	3	6. Does your school put physical education first and athletics second?
1	2	3	7. Does your school's physical education program emphasize fitness, basic skills, fun and participation rather than skill development and competition?
1	2	3	8. Are the physical education teachers in your school physically fit and involved in their own fitness program?
1	2	3	9. Do your children enjoy, speak highly of, and look forward to physical education classes?
1	2	3	10. Does your school threaten to cut physical education when budget cuts are considered?

Add your circled points for a total score.

If your score is below 24 points, follow these steps recommended by the President's Council on Physical Fitness and Sports.

1. Make sure you know what your local school code says about physical education and what is specified in state laws or regulations.
2. Determine what other school districts are doing in your area regarding physical education offerings.
3. Speak to the physical education instructor in your child's school. Hopefully, you will find him or her very cooperative and willing to answer your questions.
4. If the physical education instructor can't help, speak to the school principal.
5. If significant changes are needed in the school's priorities or scheduling, try to encourage your PTA or PTO to take up the cause of a regular physical education program.
6. If the problem is one of policy in the entire school district, take up the issue with your local Board of Education.
7. If your school is doing all it can at this time, make certain your child gets at least one half hour of vigorous physical activity every day before or after school.

Finally, I add an eighth point: If in the end your child's school doesn't respond to the need for quality physical education programs, take a radical approach. Get a note from the family physician excusing your child from physical education and enroll him in an after-school program where he will get a sound fitness education. This approach is touchy, but it gets people's attention.

Before choosing a fitness program for your child at a Y, health club, or aerobics class, try to do the following:

■ Talk to the instructor. Find out the philosophy of the instructor in terms of exercise for children. How long do the class members work out? How hard do they work out? Is the instructor aware of the psychological, physiological, and sociological aspects of children's development?
■ Observe the class in operation. Does it provide enough variety? Are the children being pushed too hard? Are the children having fun?

The quality of your children's coaching may be more difficult to evaluate. Whether he or she opts for rowing or running, you can help your child most by scouting out a good coach. "The quality of supervision in organized sports programs is crucial," says Dr. Lyle Micheli, Sports Medicine Director at Children's Hospital in Boston. "Parents need to be good customers. Look for someone who takes a positive reinforcement approach in working with the child, who tries to get the child to see himself as competing with himself, to build on his past strengths."

Talk to the coach. Ask him his philosophy. If the coach says *each* child should have a chance to play—good. You probably have a winner. Counsel your child. No matter how old your child is, keep reminding him or her that it's not winning, but playing the sport, striving for realistic goals, and giving your all that matters. This isn't just "feel good" talk, it may be the best way to make sure your small one grows into a fit adult. In other words, strive to do your best and don't worry about the competition.

The National Association for Sports and Physical Education for Youth Athletics has established guidelines called "The Youth Athlete's Bill of Rights." They require that *all* youths:

1. Participate or play.
2. Be entitled to qualified adult leadership.
3. Play as a child, not as an adult.
4. Share in leadership.
5. Participate in a safe and healthy environment.
6. Have fun.
7. Be treated with dignity.
8. Have an opportunity for success.

You and your child have a right to demand these things from your child's coach—whether he's a school coach or coach of a YMCA or after-school program. Again, be caring, committed, and united, and ask questions.

A FINAL WORD

Throughout this book I have emphasized that increased physical fitness among children may mean improved heart function, reduced body fat, and slackened heart-disease risk factors. Fitness has some other surprising benefits. Improved physical fitness may mean increased learning readiness and self-esteem, plus enhanced academic performance. Better school morale, improved class behavior, and reduced anxiety and tension have also been reported when children improve their physical fitness levels. Children between the ages of two weeks and one year old who were stimulated by exercise showed accelerated size and body weight at age one, with a greater vocabulary. At the other extreme of youth, a Florida study on college students showed that the number one alternative to drug use was physical activity and sports.

While it is true that not all of these benefits may occur with all children, it is also true that the earlier we begin improving the fitness levels of our children, the better chance they have of being not only physically healthy, but also more self-sufficient, resolute, emotionally stable, imaginative, and better prepared for the future.

Where to Get Professional Help

Amateur Athletic Union, 3400 West 86th, Indianapolis, IN 46268; (317) 872-2900.

American Academy of Pediatrics, 141 Northwest Point Road, P.O. Box 927, Elk Grove Village, IL 60007; (312) 228-5005.

American Alliance for Health, Physical Education, Recreation and Dance, 1900 Association Drive, Reston, VA 22091; (703) 476-3400.

American Anorexia/Bulimia Association, 133 Cedar Lane, Teaneck, NJ 07666; (201) 836-1800.

American College of Sports Medicine, P.O. Box 1440, Indianapolis, IN 46206-1440; (317) 637-9200.

American Health Foundation, 320 East 43rd Street, New York, NY 10017; (212) 953-1900.

American Medical Association, AMA Order Department, P.O. Box 10946, Chicago, IL 60610; (312) 645-5000. (Booklet OP 156: "Physical Activity . . . for Fitness and Health.")

Body Shop, 211 West Lake Street, Minneapolis, MN 55408; (612) 822-2000.

Consumer Information Center, Att: S. James, P.O. Box 100, Pueblo, CO 81002; (303) 948-3334. (Pamphlet 580N: "Plain Talk About Stress," single copy free.)

Feelin' Good, Fitness Finders, Inc., 133 Teft Road, P.O. Box 160, Spring Arbor, MI 49283-0160; (517) 750-1500.

Institute for Study of Youth Sports, Michigan State University, 213 I.M. Sports Circle, East Lansing, MI 48824; (517) 353-6689.

National Fitness Foundation, 2250 East Imperial Highway, Suite 412, El Segundo, CA 90245; (213) 640-0145.

National Institute for Fitness and Sport, 250 North Agnes, Indianapolis, IN 46202; (317) 274-3432.

National Youth Sports Coaches Association, 2611 Okeechobee Road, West Palm Beach, FL 33409; (305) 684-1141.

Overeaters Anonymous, World Service Office, 2190 190th Street, Torrance, CA 90504; (213) 542-8363; or contact your local unit.

President's Council on Physical Fitness & Sports, 400 South Street, SW, Washington, DC 20201; (202) 272-3421.

Shape Down Clinic, University of California—San Francisco, 55 Laguna Street, San Francisco, CA 94102; (415) 476-9000.

TOPS Club, Inc. (Take Off Pounds Sensibly, Inc.), 4575 South 5th Street, P.O. Box 07360, Milwaukee, WI 53207; (414) 482-4620; or contact your local office.

Weight Watchers, International, Jericho Atrium, 500 North Broadway, Jericho, NY 11753-2196; (516) 939-0400; or contact your local office.

YMCA of the U.S.A., 101 North Wacker Drive, Chicago, IL 60606; (312) 977-0031; or contact your local YMCA.

YWCA of the U.S.A., 726 Broadway at Waverly Street, New York, NY 10003; (212) 614-2700.

Additional Fitness Checkups for Children and Adults

Here are other fitness checkups for children. In the event children do not want to do The Run, they may do the 400-Meter Swim, Three-Mile Bike Ride, or Three-Minute Step Test.

Also included are fitness standards for adults, so Mom and Dad may compare themselves to their children's performance.

The Swim. Find a pool that has a reasonable length—25 yards or 25 meters.

Tell your children: Try to swim 440 yards (or 400 meters) as quickly as possible. If you need to stop, stop. But you may continue to walk in the water. I'll time you. When you finish, I'll compare your time with the chart.

TABLE B-1 ■ *440-Yard or 400-Meter Swim Standards (Boys)*

AGE RATING	6–7	8–9	10–11	12–13	SCORE	TIME	YOUR SCORE
Excellent	<9:10	<8:00	<7:55	<6.15	10		
Good	9:11–10:20	8:01–9:00	7:56–8:30	6:16–7:40	8		
Average	10:21–14:00	9:01–12:12	8:31–10:40	7:41–9:30	6		
Fair	14:01–15:39	12:31–14:00	10:41–11:20	9:31–10:00	4		
Poor	>15:39	>14:00	>11:20	>10:00	2		

TABLE B-2 ■ *440-Yard or 400-Meter Swim Standards (Girls)*

AGE RATING	6–7	8–9	10–11	12–13	SCORE	TIME	YOUR SCORE
Excellent	<9:45	<9:10	<9:00	<8:30	10		
Good	9:46–11:15	9:10–10:15	9:01–10:00	8:31–9:45	8		
Average	11:16–14:40	10:16–13:15	10:01–12:30	9:46–12:00	6		
Fair	14:41–16:15	13:16–15:00	12:31–13:15	12:01–12:50	4		
Poor	>16:15	>15:00	>13:15	>12:50	2		

The Bike Ride. To do the three-mile bike test, pick a course that's flat. A three-speed, ten-speed, or coaster-brake bike may be used. If a ten-speed bicycle is used, put it in the fifth gear, a three-speed in second.

Tell your children: Pedal the three miles as quickly as possible. I'll time you. Don't change gears. When you finish I'll compare your time with the chart.

Note: An exercise bicycle may be used. Set the resistance according to what you think "feels" similar to riding a bicycle on a track or level course.

TABLE B-3 ■ *Three-Mile Bike-Ride Standards (Boys)*

AGE RATING	6–7	8–9	10–11	12–13	SCORE	TIME	YOUR SCORE
Excellent	<9:45	<8:25	<8:20	<6:41	10		
Good	9:46–11:00	8:26–9:30	8:21–9:00	6:42–8:00	8		
Average	11:01–14:30	9:31–12:40	9:01–11:00	8:01–10:00	6		
Fair	14:31–16:15	12:41–14:25	11:01–11:40	10:01–10:30	4		
Poor	>16:15	>14:25	>11:41	>10:31	2		

TABLE B-4 ■ *Three-Mile Bike-Ride Standards (Girls)*

AGE RATING	6–7	8–9	10–11	12–13	SCORE	TIME	YOUR SCORE
Excellent	<10:30	<9:40	<9:45	<9:05	10		
Good	10:31–12:00	9:41–11:00	9:46–10:50	9:06–10:15	8		
Average	12:01–15:30	11:01–14:00	10:51–13:15	10:16–12:35	6		
Fair	15:31–17:00	14:01–15:25	13:16–14:00	12:36–13:30	4		
Poor	>17:00	>15:25	>14:00	>13:30	2		

Cardiovascular Fitness Test

The Step Test. The Step Test measures the heart's ability to recover after endurance-type activities. A quick recovery indicates an efficient heart. An efficient heart may reduce the risk of heart disease.

Tell your children:

- I want you to step up and down on this bench (or a stack of neatly tied newspapers; either should be 12 inches).
- Take 24 steps per minute. That's one step every 2.5 seconds. I'll count your steps. (A metronome may be used, you can count out

a cadence, or put your voice on a tape recorder.) Step with each count. A cycle consists of stepping first with the right foot on the bench, then the left. Then returning the right, then left foot to the floor.

■ After stepping for three minutes stop and rest for exactly five seconds. Then I'll take your pulse for one minute. I'll compare your rate with the chart.

TABLE B-5 ■ *Three-Minute Step-Test Standards*

AGE SEX RATING	6–7 M	F	8–9 M	F	10–11 M	F	12–13 M	F	SCORE	HEART RATE	YOUR SCORE
Excellent	106*	110*	104*	108*	94*	99*	90*	97*	10		
Good	107–116	111–119	105–112	109–115	95–103	100–110	91–100	98–105	8		
Average	117–126	120–129	113–122	116–129	104–110	111–120	101–110	106–118	6		
Fair	127–136	130–139	123–130	130–137	111–124	121–130	111–124	119–128	4		
Poor	137+	140+	130+	138+	125+	131+	125+	129+	2		

* Or below

FITNESS STANDARDS FOR ADULTS

Muscle Fitness

Curl-Ups. Do exercise as described on page 84.

TABLE B-6 ▪ *Curl-Ups Test Standards (number completed in one minute)*

AGE	19–29		30–39		40–49		50–59		60–69		SCORE
SEX	M	F	M	F	M	F	M	F	M	F	
RATING											
Excellent	51+	46+	46+	41+	41+	36+	36+	31+	31+	26+	5
Good	43–50	38–45	35–45	30–40	30–40	25–35	25–35	20–30	20–30	15–25	4
Average	30–42	25–37	25–34	20–29	20–29	15–24	16–24	11–19	13–19	8–14	3
Fair	20–29	15–24	15–24	10–19	10–19	8–14	8–15	6–10	6–12	3–7	2
Poor	0–20	0–14	0–14	0–9	0–10	0–8	0–7	0–6	0–6	0–2	1

Push-Ups. Do exercise as described on page 83.

TABLE B-7 ▪ *Push-Ups Test Standards (number completed in one minute)*

AGE	19–29		30–39		40–49		50–59		60–69		SCORE
SEX	M	F	M	F	M	F	M	F	M	F	
RATING											
Excellent	51+	46+	46+	41+	41+	36+	36+	31+	31+	26+	5
Good	45–50	34–45	35–45	25–40	30–39	20–35	25–35	15–30	20–30	10–25	4
Average	34–44	17–33	25–34	12–24	20–29	8–19	15–24	6–14	10–19	3–9	3
Fair	20–33	6–16	15–24	4–11	12–19	3–7	8–14	2–5	5–9	1–2	2
Poor	0–19	0–5	0–14	0–3	0–11	0–2	0–7	0–1	0–4	0	1

Flexibility

Sit-and-Reach. Do exercise as described on page 25.

TABLE B-8 ■ *Sit-and-Reach Test Standards*

ALL AGE GROUPS RATING		FITNESS SCORE
Excellent	Palms flat against the wall	5
Good	Knuckles touch the wall	4
Average	Fingertips touch toes or wall	3
Fair	Fingertips are 1 to 3 inches from toes	2
Poor	Fingertips are 4 or more inches from toes	1

Cardiovascular Fitness

Three-Minute Step Test. Do exercise as described on pages 187–188.

TABLE B-9 ■ *Three-Minute Step-Test Norms (Heart Rate)*

AGE SEX RATING	14–29		30–39		40–49		50–59		60 AND OVER		FITNESS SCORE
	M	F	M	F	M	F	M	F	M	F	
Excellent	<74	<79	<77	<83	<79	<87	<85	<91	<89	<94	10
Good	75–90	80–101	78–99	84–105	80–100	88–108	86–105	92–113	90–108	95–117	8
Average	91–100	102–119	100–109	106–122	101–112	109–118	106–115	114–123	109–118	118–127	6
Fair	101–120	120–133	110–125	123–135	113–125	119–130	116–130	124–136	119–130	128–140	4
Poor	121+	134+	126+	136+	126+	131+	131+	137+	131+	141+	2

Fat/Weight

This measurement determines how much fat is on the adult body.

Women: Measure the circumference of your hips at the widest part. Then locate your hip girth and your height in inches on the chart* below. A line connecting them will indicate your percent of body fat, which should be no more than 23 percent.

Men: Measure the circumference of your waist at the navel. Then use chart as above to determine body fat. It should be no more than 15 percent.

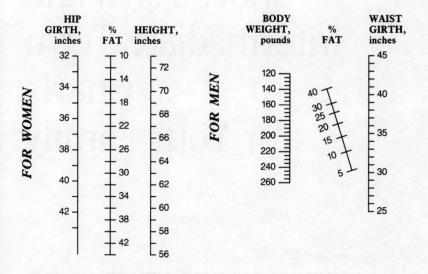

* Jack Wilmore, Director, Adult Fitness Program, University of Texas.

APPENDIX **C**

Short-Term and Intermediate-Term Charts for Your Family

Short-Term Goal Chart

SHORT-TERM GOAL	OBSTACLES	HOW TO GET AROUND	DATE ACCOM-PLISHED	REWARD

Short-Term Goal Chart

SHORT-TERM GOAL	OBSTACLES	HOW TO GET AROUND	DATE ACCOM-PLISHED	REWARD

Short-Term Goal Chart

SHORT-TERM GOAL	OBSTACLES	HOW TO GET AROUND	DATE ACCOM-PLISHED	REWARD

Intermediate Goal Chart

INTER-MEDIATE GOAL	OBSTACLES	HOW TO GET AROUND	DATE ACCOM-PLISHED	REWARD

Intermediate Goal Chart

INTER-MEDIATE GOAL	OBSTACLES	HOW TO GET AROUND	DATE ACCOM-PLISHED	REWARD

Intermediate Goal Chart

INTER- MEDIATE GOAL	OBSTACLES	HOW TO GET AROUND	DATE ACCOM- PLISHED	REWARD

Home Gym Equipment

Before buying any exercise equipment recognize that equipment is merely a crutch. You can become fit with walking, running, and calisthenics. Equipment is nice and helpful, but don't be lulled into thinking the equipment will get you into shape. You must do the work.

Before purchasing, consider the following:

Stationary bicycles. Choose a unit with a sturdy frame. The wheel should be heavy to provide a smooth effect as you pedal, with no jerkiness or wobble. Make sure the seat is comfortable and adjustable.

Variable resistance is important. You should be able to increase or decrease pedal pressure to suit your exercise needs. It is best if the resistance device is calibrated so you can adjust resistance precisely.

A speedometer, odometer, and a timer help guarantee that you can get the amount of exercise you want. The more sophisticated units tell you, your doctor, or your fitness leader exactly how much exercise you are getting in terms of internationally recognized workload standards. The readings are in watts, newton meters (NM), or kilogram meters (Kgm).

Rowing machines. Look for durability, a smooth pattern as you row, hydraulic levers, adjustable tension, and a sturdy seat. The Concept II operates on different principles. Expensive ($600) but simulates real rowing.

Treadmills. Stay away from nonmotorized treadmills, unless you plan only to walk. Even then you must be cautious that the rollers are durable, and expect a hot foot if you walk rapidly or for long periods of time. As a rule, electric treadmills are pretty good. Most are over $1,000. Before purchasing, run for at least five minutes on it. If you experience a pause, delay, or jerkiness of the belt, you probably need a heavier model to adequately support your weight. The "mill" should have a minimum of two speeds and a manual or electric height adjustment. A handrail is standard. The height of the treadmill is a consideration. If the treadmill belt is more than eight inches off the floor, you may have a problem with ceiling height.

Resistance machines. Many machines are available. Look for one that allows you to add more weight as your muscle fitness improves. Ten-pound increases are the maximum. A multipurpose machine (one on which you can exercise the upper, middle, and lower thirds of your body) is best.

Passive equipment—the no-sweat exercise. Exercise equipment works in one of two ways: 1) active—you work on the machine; or 2) passive—the machine works on you.

Passive exercise equipment has little physical fitness value; it doesn't improve cardiovascular and muscular fitness and suppleness. Passive machines may relax you and make you feel like a million bucks, but as the American Medical Association's Committee on Exercise and Physical Fitness has said, "Effortless exercise [passive] . . . cannot benefit a person in any magical way." In short, if you are going to benefit from exercise, you must put effort into it. Passive exercise cannot help you become fit, nor will it roll off the fat. If you don't have to exert effort on the machine, forget it. Sample passive equipment includes: belt vibrators, massage rollers, massage machines and accessories, massage stimulators, sauna shorts, saunas, hot tubs, whirlpools, sensory isolation tanks, reducing machines (worthless), and suntanning equipment.

198 ■ *APPENDIX D*

A third type of product might be called mild exercise equipment. Here the exercise demand is very slight and *effective only for the ill or infirm*. These include hip-pedacycles, twist boards, and rubber stretchers.

Bibliography

Adams, F. H., et al. "The Physical Working Capacity of Normal School Children: California." *Pediatrics*, 28: 55, 1961.

Allen, R. E., and C. Kraft. *Handbook for Cultural Analysis and Change.* Morristown, N.J.: HRI Press, 1980.

American Alliance for Health, Physical Education, Recreation and Dance. "Summary of Findings from National Children and Youth Fitness Study II." *Journal of Physical Education, Recreation and Dance*, 58: 49, 1987.

American Alliance for Health, Physical Education, Recreation and Dance. "Summary of Findings from National Children and Youth Fitness Study." *Journal of Physical Education, Recreation and Dance*, 56: 45, 1985.

American Alliance for Health, Physical Education, Recreation and Dance. *Health Related Physical Fitness Test Manual.* Reston, Va.: AAHPERD, 1980.

American College of Sports Medicine Position Stands and Opinion Statements, Indianapolis, Indiana. "The Recommended Quantity and Quality of Exercise for Developing and Maintaining Fitness in Healthy Adults," 1975–83; and "Physical Fitness in Children and Youth," 1988.

Astrand, P. O., and K. Rodahl. *Textbook of Work Physiology.* New York: McGraw-Hill, 1970.

Bailer, I. "Conceptualization of Success and Failure in Mentally Retarded and Normal Children." *Journal of Personality*, 29: 303, 1961.

Bailey, D. A. "Exercise, Fitness and Physical Education for the Growing Child—a Concern." *Canadian Journal of Public Health*, 64: 421–430, 1973.

Bailey, D. A., and R. L. Mirwald. "A Children's Test of Fitness." *Pediatric Work Physiology*. Basel, Switzerland: S. Karger, 1978: 56–64.

Bailey, D. A., et al. "The Influence of Exercise, Physical Activity, and Athletic Performance on the Dynamics of Human Growth." In F. Falkner, ed. *Human Growth*, Vol. II, 1978–79, pp. 475–501.

Bailey, D. A., et al. "Size Dissociation of Maximal Aerobic Power During Growth in Boys." *Pediatric Work Physiology*. Basel, Switzerland: S. Karger, 1978: 140–51.

Bar-Or, O., ed. *Pediatric Work Physiology*. Proceedings of the Fourth International Symposium. Wingate Institute, Israel, 1982.

Beardall, S. "Today's Children Fatter, Sicker and More Disturbed." *The Times*, London, England, November 9, 1985.

Berenson, G. S., et al. "Cardiovascular Disease Risk Factor Variables at the Preschool Age: The Bogalusa Heart Study." *Circulation*, 57 (3): 603–12, March 1978.

Berenson, G. S., et al. *Cardiovascular Risk Factors in Children*. New York: Oxford University Press, 1980.

Beunen, G., et al. "Age of Menarche and Motor Performance in Girls Aged 11 Through 18." *Pediatric Work Physiology*. Basel, Switzerland: S. Karger, 1978: 118–23.

Boileau, R. A., et al. "Comparison of Three Treadmill Walking Tests to Evaluate Physiological Responses to Exercise of Young Children." *Annali Dell' Isef* III (2), December 1984.

Boileau, R. A., et al. "Exercise and Body Composition of Children and Youth." *Scandanavian Journal of Sports Science* 7 (1): 17–27, 1985.

Boileau, R. A., et al. "Hydration of the Fat-free Body in Children During Maturation." *Human Biology*, 56 (4): 651–66, December 1984.

Borms, J., and M. Hebbelinck. "Introduction." *Pediatric Work Physiology*. Basel, Switzerland: S. Karger, 1978: 1–28.

Bradfield, R. B., et al. "Energy Expenditures and Heart Rates of Cambridge Boys at School." *The American Journal of Clinical Nutrition*, 24: 1461–66, December 1971.

Breckenridge, M. E., and E. L. Vincent. *Child Development*. Philadelphia: W. B. Saunders Co., 1966.

Briggs, T. W. "Kids and Sports: The Playing's the Thing." *USA Today,* April 25, 1988, 1D.

Brinkman, J. R., and T. A. Hoskins. "Physical Conditioning and Altered Self-concept." In "Rehabilitated Hemiplegic Patients," *Physical Therapy,* 59: 859, 1979.

Brooks, G. A., and T. D. Fahey. *Exercise Physiology: Human Bioenergetics and Its Applications.* New York: John Wiley & Sons, 1984.

Brownell, K. D. *The LEARN Manual for Weight Control.* Philadelphia: Kelly D. Brownell, Ph.D., 1985.

Brownell, K. D. "Making It Permanent." *The Turnaround Lifestyle System,* Campbell's Institute for Health and Fitness. Camden, N.J.: Campbell Soup Company, 1984.

Canadian Association for Health, Physical Education and Recreation. *The CAHPER Fitness-Performance Test Manual.* Ontario, Canada, 1966.

Caplan, T., and F. Caplan. *The Early Childhood Years: The 2 to 6 Year Old.* New York: Bantam Books, 1983.

Carey, J., et al. "America's Kids: Why They're Out of Shape." *Newsweek,* April 1, 1985, pp. 84–85.

Chausow, S. A., et al. "Metabolic and Cardiovascular Responses of Children During Prolonged Physical Activity." *Research Quarterly,* 55 (1): 1–7, 1984.

Clarke, H. H. *Physical and Motor Tests in the Medford Boy's Growth Study.* Englewood Cliffs, N.J.: Prentice-Hall, Inc., 1971.

Committee on Sports Medicine. American Academy of Pediatrics. "Sports Medicine: Health Care for Youth Athletes." Evanston, Ill.: American Academy of Pediatrics, 1983.

Connor, W. E. "Cross-cultural Studies of Diet and Plasma Lipids and Lipoproteins." In *Childhood Prevention of Atherosclerosis and Hypertension,* R. M. Lauer and R. B. Shekelle, eds. New York: Raven Press, 1980.

Cooper, K. H. *The Aerobics Way.* New York: M. Evans, 1977.

Cooper, K. H., et al. "Physical Fitness versus Selected Coronary Risk Factors: A Cross-sectional Study." *Journal of the American Medical Association,* 236: 166, 1976.

Coopersmith, S. *The Antecedents of Self-Esteem.* San Francisco: W. H. Freeman and Co., 1967.

Coronary Heart Disease in Adults. United States 1960–62. U.S. Department of Health, Education and Welfare, Public Health Service. Data from the National Survey, Vital and Health Statistics 11, No. 10, 1965.

Cratty, B. J. *Movement Behavior and Motor Learning.* Philadelphia: Lea & Febiger, 1964.

Cumming, G. R., and R. Keynes. "A Fitness Performance Test for School Children and Its Correlation with Physical Working Capacity and Maximal Oxygen Uptake." *Canadian Medical Association Journal.* Vol. 96, May 6, 1967, pp. 1262–69.

Cumming, G. R., et al. "Failure of School Physical Education to Improve Cardiorespiratory Fitness." *Canadian Medical Association Journal,* Vol. 101, July 26, 1969, pp. 69–73.

Cureton, T. K. *Improving the Physical Fitness of Youth.* Monographs of the Society for Research in Child Development, 29: 4, 1964.

Cureton, T. K. Personal communication. 1976 and 1981.

Deitz, W. H. "Do We Fatten Our Children at the Television Set? Obesity and Television Viewing in Children and Adolescents." *Pediatrics,* 75: 807, 1985.

Deitz, W. H., and J. E. Gordon. "Obesity in Infants, Children and Adolescents in the United States." *Nutrition Research,* 1: 193, 1981.

Dill, D. B. "Effects of Physical Strain and Health Activities on the Heart and Circulation." *American Heart Journal,* 23: 441, 1942.

Drash, A. "Atherosclerosis, Cholesterol, and the Pediatrician." *Journal of Pediatrics,* 80: 693, 1972.

Drash, A., and F. Hengstenberg. "The Identification of Risk Factors in Normal Children in the Development of Arteriosclerosis." *Annals of Clinical Laboratory Science,* 2 (5): 348–59, 1972.

Driscoll, D. J. "Cardiovascular Evaluation of the Child and Adolescent Before Participation in Sports." *Mayo Clinic Proceedings,* 60: 867–873, 1985.

Dyer, W. W. *What Do You Really Want for Your Children?* New York: William Morrow & Company, Inc., 1985.

Eggen, D. A., and L. A. Solberg. "Variation of Atherosclerosis with Age." *Laboratory Investigation,* 18: 571, 1968.

Ekblom, B. "Effect of Physical Training in Adolescent Boys." *Journal of Applied Psychology,* 27 (3): 350–55, September 1969.

Endres, J. B., and R. E. Rockwell. *Food, Nutrition, and the Young Child.* St. Louis: C.V. Mosby Company, 1980.

Eriksson, B. O. "Physical Training, Oxygen Supply and Muscle Metabolism in 11-13-Year-Old Boys." *Acta Physiologica Scandinavica.* trans. W. P. Michael. Stockholm, 1972, pp. 2–48.

Feinsilber, M., and W. Mead. *American Averages.* Garden City, N.Y.: Dolphin Books, 1980.

Fiedler, L., et al. *Progress Report and Comparison Analysis Health Attitudes Survey, Coronary Heart Disease Risk Factors in Children.* Office of Educational Resources and Research, Department of Postgraduate Medicine and Health Professions Education, Technical Memo #81.4. Ann Arbor, Mich.: The University of Michigan Medical Center, G-111 Towsley Center, 1981.

"Finds Children Are 'Enormously' Competent at Self-care." *Pediatric News,* 18 (10): 67, October 1984.

Fohlen, L., et al. "Body Dimensions and Exercise Performance in Anorexia Nervosa Patients." *Pediatric Work Physiology.* Basel, Switzerland: S. Karger, 1978: 102–107.

Forbes, G. B. "Body Composition in Adolescence." In F. Falkner, ed. *Human Growth,* Vol. II, 1978–79, pp. 239–67.

Friedman, G. "A Pediatrician Looks at Risk Factors in Atherosclerotic Heart Disease." *Clinical Research,* 20: 250, 1972.

Friend, T. "Cholesterol, Fat Creep Up on Our Kids." *USA Today,* May 26, 1988, p. 1A.

Gergen, K. J. *The Concept of Self.* New York: Holt, Rinehart and Winston, 1971.

Gilliam, T. B., and P. S. Freedson. "Effects of a Twelve-week School Physical Fitness Program on Peak VO_2, Body Composition and Blood Lipids in 7 to 9 Year Old Children." *International Journal of Sports Medicine,* 1: 78, 1980.

Gilliam, T. B., et al. "Exercise Programs for Children: A Way to Prevent Heart Disease." *The Physician and Sports Medicine,* 10: 96, 1982.

Gilliam, T. B., et al. "Prevalence of Coronary Heart Disease Risk Factors in Active Children, 7 to 12 Years of Age." *Medicine and Science in Sports,* 9: 21, 1977.

Golding, L., et al. *The Y's Way to Physical Fitness.* Chicago: National Board of YMCA, 1982.

Gordon, T., et al. "High-density Lipoprotein as a Protective Factor Against Coronary Heart Disease." *American Journal of Medicine,* 62: 293, 1976.

Gortmaker, L., et al. "Increasing Pediatric Obesity in the United States." *American Journal of Disease Control,* 141: 535, 1987.

Goulian, L. "Fitness Is Child's Play, Too." *Sports, Inc.*, January 25, 1988, p. 46.

Guilford, J. P. *Fundamental Statistics in Psychology and Education.* New York: McGraw-Hill, 1956.

Hackman, E. M. "Four-Star Fast Foods." *Shape*, August 1987, p. 42.

Hackman, E. M. "Picky Eaters." *Shape*, February 1987, p. 26.

Haney, D. Q. "Study Links Cholesterol, Artery Damage in Childhood." *The Ledger*, January 16, 1986, p. 9A.

Hansen, B. C., ed. *Controversies in Obesity.* New York: Praeger Publishers, 1983.

Harris, L. J., et al. *Algorithms for Health Planners: Heart Attack Mortality,* Vol. 4. Santa Monica: The Rand Corporation, 1977.

Haskell, W., et al., eds. *Nutrition and Athletic Performance.* Proceedings of the Conference on Nutritional Determinants in Athletic Performance. San Francisco: September 1981.

Healthy People. The Surgeon General's Report on Health Promotion and Disease Prevention 1979. U.S. Department of Health, Education and Welfare, Public Health Service, 1979.

Healthy People. The Surgeon General's Report on Health Promotion and Disease Prevention—Background Papers 1979, "Tobacco, Alcohol and Drug Abuse: Onset and Prevention." U.S. Department of Health, Education and Welfare, Public Health Service, 1979, p. 197.

Healy, M., and S. A. Stewart. "Parents Try to Spark a Junior Fitness Craze." *USA Today*, Thursday, March 20, 1986, p. 1D.

Hebbelinck, M. "Methods of Biological Maturity Assessment." *Pediatric Work Physiology.* Basel, Switzerland: S. Karger, 1978: 108–17.

Hellmich, N. "Parents Set Tone for Fitness." *USA Today*, December 1, 1987, p. 4D.

Henry, M. M. "Reduce Junk Food in School Cafeterias, Dietitian Advises." *The Philadelphia Inquirer*, February 18, 1986, p. 7B.

Holliday, M. A. "Body Composition and Energy Needs During Growth." In F. Falkner, ed. *Human Growth*, Vol. II, 1978–79, pp. 117–37.

Hurych, J., et al. "Precursors of Atherosclerosis in Schoolchildren." *Cor Vasa* (1981), 23 (3): 161–71.

Ikeda, J. *Change Your Habits to Change Your Shape.* Palo Alto, Cal.: Bull Publishing Co., 1978.

Ismail, A. H., and L. E. Trachtman. "Jogging the Imagination." *Psychology Today*, 7: 79, 1973.

Jackson, A. S., and A. E. Coleman. "Validation of Distance Run Tests for Elementary School Children." *Research Quarterly*, 47: 86, 1976.

Jacobson, M. F. *The Complete Eater's Digest and Nutrition Scoreboard*. Garden City, N.Y.: Anchor Press, 1974.

Jenkins, G. G., et al. *Guidebook for Health and Safety for Teen-Agers*. Chicago: Scott, Foresman and Co., 1962.

Kannel, W., et al. "Serum Cholesterol, Lipoproteins and the Risk of Coronary Heart Disease." *Annals of Internal Medicine*, 74: 1, 1971.

Kannel, W. B. "Coronary Risk Factors, II: Prospects for Prevention of Atherosclerosis in the Young." *New Zealand Journal of Medicine* (1976), 6 (5): 410–19.

Kannel, W. B. *Handbook of Coronary Risk Probability*. New York: American Heart Association, 1972.

Kannel, W. B., and T. R. Dawber. "Atherosclerosis as a Pediatric Problem." *Journal of Pediatrics*, 80: 544, 1972.

Kelly, M., and E. P. Larsons. *The Mother's Almanac*. Garden City, N.Y.: Doubleday & Company, Inc., 1975.

Kemper, H. C. G., et al. "Investigation into the Effects of Two Extra Physical Education Lessons per Week During One School Year upon the Physical Development of 12- and 13-Year-Old Boys." *Pediatric Work Physiology*. Basel, Switzerland: S. Karger, 1978: 159–72.

Kirschenbaum, J., and R. Sullivan. "Hold on There, America." *Sports Illustrated*, 58 (5): 60–73, February 7, 1983.

Knuttgen, H. G. "Comparison of Fitness of Danish and American School Children." *Research Quarterly*, 32 (2): 190–96, 1961.

Kobayashi, K., et al. "Aerobic Power as Related to Body Growth and Training in Japanese Boys: A Longitudinal Study." *The American Physiological Society*, 1978, pp. 666–72.

Koch, G. "Muscle Blood Flow in Prepubertal Boys." *Pediatric Work Physiology*. Basel, Switzerland: S. Karger, 1978: 39–46.

Krahenbuhl, G. S., et al. "Field Estimation of VO_2 Max in Children Eight Years of Age." *Medicine and Science in Sports*, 9: 37, 1977.

Krassean, B. "TV and the Fat Kid: Small-Fry Couch Potatoes on the Rise." *Jackson Citizen Patriot*, Tuesday, June 30, 1987, p. 1B.

Kuntzleman, C. T. *The Beat Goes On*. Spring Arbor, Mich.: Arbor Press, 1980.

Kuntzleman, C. T. *Color Me Red!* Spring Arbor, Mich.: Arbor Press, 1977.

Kuntzleman, C. T. "Feelin' Good" film. Spring Arbor, Mich.: Fitness Finders, Inc., 1982.

Kuntzleman, C. T. *Fitness Discovery Activities*. Spring Arbor, Mich.: Arbor Press, 1978.

Kuntzleman, C. T. *Heartbeat*. Spring Arbor, Mich.: Arbor Press, 1977.

Kuntzleman, C. T. "The Reader's Digest Family Fitness Guide." *Reader's Digest*, Pleasantville, N.Y., January 1986.

Kuntzleman, C. T. *Values Strategies for Fitness*. Spring Arbor, Mich.: Arbor Press, 1978.

Kuntzleman, C. T. *The Well Family Book*. San Bernardino, Cal.: Here's Life Publishers, 1985.

Kuntzleman, C. T., and D. Drake. *The Feelin' Good Youth Fitness Report*. Spring Arbor, Mich.: Fitness Finders, Inc., 1984.

Kuntzleman, C. T., and D. Runyon. *Parent's Guide to Feelin' Good*. Spring Arbor, Mich.: Arbor Press, 1982.

Lauer, R. M., et al. "The Coronary Heart Disease Risk Factors in School Children: The Muscatine Study." *Journal of Pediatrics*, 86: 697, 1975.

Leveille, G. A. *The Setpoint Diet*. New York: Ballantine Books, 1985.

Levy, J. *The Baby Exercise Book*. New York: Pantheon Books, 1975.

Levy, R. I., et al., eds. *Nutrition, Lipids, and Coronary Heart Disease: A Global View*. Vol. I, *Nutrition in Health and Disease*. New York: Raven Press, 1979.

Lewis, C. E., and M. A. Lewis. "Child-initiated Health Care." *The Journal of School Health*, March 1980, pp. 144–48.

Lewis, M. A. "Child-initiated Care." *American Journal of Nursing*, 74 (4): 652–55, April 1974.

Linde, L. M. "An Appraisal of Exercise Fitness Tests." *Pediatrics*, 32: 656, 1963.

The Lipid Research Clinics Population Studies Data Book. Vol. 1, *The Prevalence Study*. U.S. Department of Health and Human Services, Public Health Service, National Institutes of Health, 80–1527, 1980.

The Lipid Research Clinics Population Studies Data Book. Vol. II, *The Prevalence Study—Nutrient Intake*. U.S. Department of Health and Human Services, Public Health Service, National Institutes of Health, 82–2014, 1982.

Londe, S., et al. "Hypertension in Apparently Normal Children." *Journal of Pediatrics*, 78: 569, 1971.

Luyken, R., et al. "Studies of Adolescents in the Netherlands with Special Reference to Training." In *Nutrient Requirements in Adolescence*, J. I. McKigney and H. N. Munro, eds. Cambridge, Mass.: MIT Press, 1976.

Magill, R. A., et al., eds. *Children in Sport*. Champaign, Ill.: Human Kinetics Publishers, Inc., 1982.

Marmot, M. G. "Epidemiological Basis for the Prevention of Coronary Heart Disease." *Bulletin WHO*, 57: 331, 1979.

Mayer, J. *Overweight: Causes, Cost and Control*. Englewood Cliffs, N.J.: Prentice-Hall, Inc., 1968.

McArdle, W. D., et al. *Exercise Physiology*. Philadelphia: Lea & Febiger, 1981.

McDonough, J. R., and R. A. Bruce. "Maximal Exercise Testing in Assessing Cardiovascular Function." *The Journal of the South Carolina Medical Association*, 65: 26, 1969.

McGill, H. C., Jr. "Morphologic Development of the Atherosclerotic Plaque." In *Childhood Prevention of Atherosclerosis and Hypertension*, R. M. Lauer and R. B. Shekelle, eds. New York: Raven Press, 1980.

Mellin, L. *Shapedown*. San Francisco: Balboa Publishing, 1983.

Morgan, W. P. "Anxiety Reduction Following Acute Exercise." *Psychiatric Annals*, 9: 141, 1979.

Mroczek, W. J. "High School Health Curriculum: A Neglected Medical Resource." *American Heart Journal*, 92: 271, 1976.

National Academy of Sciences and National Research Council. *Nutritional Review*, 38, August 1980.

National Association for Sport and Physical Education. *Adolescence*. Reston, Va.: AAHPERD, 1981.

National Association for Sport and Physical Education. *Childhood*. Reston, Va.: AAHPERD, 1981.

National Association for Sport and Physical Education. *Early Childhood*. Reston, Va.: AAHPERD, 1981.

National Heart, Lung, and Blood Institute. *Cardiovascular Profile of 15,000 Children of School Age in Three Communities 1971–1975*. Department of Health, Education and Welfare, 78–1477. Washington, D.C., 1978.

Natow, A., and J. A. Heslin. *No-Nonsense Nutrition for Kids*. New York: Pocket Books, 1985.

Neimark, J. *American Health*, December 1984, 3 (9): 14.

Newman, W. P., and J. P. Strong. "Natural History, Geographic Pathology, and Pediatric Aspects of Atherosclerosis." In *Atherosclerosis: Its Pediatric Aspects*, W.B. Strong, ed. New York: Grune & Stratton, 1978.

Nowicki, S., Jr., and B. R. Stuckland. "A Locus of Control Scale for Children." *Journal of Consulting and Clinical Psychology*, 40: 148, 1973.

Nutrition and Your Health: Dietary Guidelines for Americans. Washington, D.C.: U.S. Department of Agriculture (Office of Governmental and Public Affairs), 1980.

Oliver, W. J., et al. "Blood Pressure, Sodium Intake, and Sodium-related Hormones in the Yanomamo Indians, a 'No-salt' culture." *Circulation*, 52: 146, 1975.

Parcel, G. S., et al. "School Promotion of Healthful Diet and Exercise Behavior: An Integration of Organizational Change and Social Learning Theory Interventions." *Journal of School Health*, 57: 150, 1987.

Parizkova, J. "Total Body Fat and Skin-fold Thickness in Children." *Metabolism*, 10: 794, 1961.

Pate, R. R. "Exercise and Coronary Heart Disease Risk: Pediatric Implications." In *Exercise and Heart Diseases: Theory and Application to Public School Physical Education*, W. G. Squires and G. J. Holland, eds. Reston, Va.: AAHPERD, 1980.

Piers, E., and D. Harris. *The Piers-Harris Children's Self-Concept Scale.* Counselor Recording and Tests, Box 6184, Acklen Stations, Nashville, Tenn., 1969.

Progress Report Health Attitude Survey. Child Exercise and Coronary Heart Disease Risk Factors in Children. Office of Educational Resources and Research, Department of Postgraduate Medicine and Health Professions Education, Technical Memo #80.1. Ann Arbor, Mich.: The University of Michigan Medical Center, G-111 Towsley Center, 1980.

Rarick, G. L., ed. *Physical Activity: Human Growth and Development.* New York: Academic Press, 1973.

Rayner, C. *The Body Book.* London: Piccolo Picture Books, 1978.

Recommended Daily Allowances, 9th ed. National Academy of Sciences, 1980.

Rhoads, C., et al. "Serum Lipoproteins and Coronary Heart Disease in a

Population Study of Hawaii Japanese Men." *New England Journal of Medicine*, 294: 293, 1976.

Rowland, T. W. "Motivational Factors in Exercise Training Programs for Children." *The Physician and Sports Medicine*, 14 (2): 122–26, 1986.

Seals, D. R., and J. M. Hagberg. "Exercise Training and Human Hypertension." *Medicine and Science in Sports and Exercise*, 16 (3): 210, 1984.

Seely, J. E., et al. "Heart and Lung Function at Rest and During Exercise in Adolescence." *Journal of Applied Psychology*, 36 (1): 34–40, January 1974.

Shephard, R. J., et al. "Curricular Time for Physical Education." *Journal of Physical Education, Recreation and Dance*, 53: 19, 1982.

Shephard, R. J., et al. "The Working Capacity of Toronto Schoolchildren, Part II." *Canadian Medical Association Journal*, 100: 705–14, April 19, 1969.

Sonstroem, R. J. "Exercise and Self-esteem." In *Exercise and Sport Sciences Reviews*, 12: 123, 1984.

Sprynarova, S., et al. "Development of the Functional Capacity and Body Composition of Boy and Girl Swimmers Aged 12–15 Years." *Pediatric Work Physiology*. Basel, Switzerland: S. Karger, 1978: 32–38.

Srinivasan, S. Z., et al. "Serum Lipoprotein Profile in Children from a Biracial Community—Bogalusa Heart Study." *Circulation*, 54: 309, 1976.

Strong. W. B. "Is Atherosclerosis a Pediatric Problem? An Overview." In *Atherosclerosis: Its Pediatric Aspects*, W. B. Strong, ed. New York: Grune and Stratton, 1979.

Sullivan, S. A. *The Father's Almanac*. Garden City, N.Y.: Doubleday & Company, Inc., 1980.

Sutton-Smith, B. "The Child at Play." *Psychology Today*, 19 (10): 64–65, 68, October 1985.

Taylor, H. L., et al. "The Effects of Bed Rest on Cardiovascular Function and Work Performance." *Journal of Applied Physiology*, 2: 223, 1949.

Thoren, C. "Working Capacity in Anorexia Nervosa." *Pediatric Work Physiology*. Basel, Switzerland: S. Karger, 1978: 89–95.

U.S. Department of Health, Education, and Welfare. *Infant Care*. Children's Bureau Publication #8—1963. Washington, D.C.: U.S. Government Printing Office, 1967.

Vajda, A. S., and M. Hebbelinck. "Secular Growth Trend Data in Belgian Populations since 1840." *Pediatric Work Physiology.* Basel, Switzerland: S. Karger, 1978: 134–39.

Van Wieringen, J. C. "Secular Growth Changes." In F. Falkner, ed. *Human Growth,* Vol. II, 1978–79, pp. 239–54.

Vital Statistics Report. NCHS Growth Charts, 1976. National Center for Health Statistics. Vol. 25 (No. 3), Supplement June 22, 1976.

Voller, R. D., and W. B. Strong. "Pediatric Aspects of Atherosclerosis." *American Heart Journal,* June 1981, pp. 815–36.

Voors, A. W., et al. "Studies of Blood Pressure in Children Ages 5–14 Years in a Total Biracial Community: The Bogalusa Heart Study." *Circulation,* 54: 319, 1976.

Vrijens, J. "Muscle Strength Development in the Pre- and Post-pubescent Age." *Pediatric Work Physiology.* Basel, Switzerland: S. Karger, 1978: 152–58.

Webber, L. S., et al. "Tracking of Cardiovascular Disease Risk Factor Variables in School-age Children." *Journal of Chronic Diseases,* 36 (9): 647–60, 1983.

White, C. W., et al. "Iowa Cardiovascular Health Knowledge Test." *Circulation,* 56: 480, 1977.

White, C. W., et al. "The Status of Cardiovascular Health Knowledge Among Sixth, Seventh and Eighth Grade Children." *Circulation,* 56: 480, 1977.

Wilmore, J. H., and J. J. McNamara. "Prevalence of Coronary Heart Disease Risk Factors in Boys, 8 to 12 Years of Age." *Journal of Pediatrics,* 84 (4): 527, 1974.

Wilson, N. L., ed. *Obesity.* Philadelphia: F. A. Davis Company, 1969.

Wynder, E. L. "Conference on Blood Lipids in Children: Optimal Levels for Early Prevention of Coronary Artery Disease." *Preventive Medicine,* 12: 741, 1983.

Young, G. "Children Need More Exercise." *Jackson Citizen Patriot,* Friday, November 15, 1985, p. B-3.

Index

ABOUT THE AUTHOR

Charles T. Kuntzleman, the distinguished author of many publications on health, has been featured on nationwide television and radio. He has conducted over 500 health and fitness seminars worldwide, and acted as a consultant or spokesperson for many leading organizations, including the National Board of YMCAs, *Reader's Digest* and *Consumer Guide*. A former small college All-American in football, a football coach and college professor, Dr. Kuntzleman developed the highly successful Feelin' Good Program for children, in which over two million kids nationwide participated. The author is a recipient of the prestigious Healthy American Fitness Leader Award. His wife and five children are very active in running, biking and swimming.